THERAPY WITH TREATMENT RESISTANT FAMILIES: A CONSULTATION-CRISIS INTERVENTION MODEL

William George McCown, PhD
Judith Johnson, PhD
and Associates

SOME ADVANCE REVIEWS

"In a field flooded with contributions, this book makes a solid and unique impact. This state-of-the-art compendium blends substantive models of family stress, coping, dysfunction, approaches to assessment, and avenues of intervention into a highly effective, practical strategy for dealing with the most difficult of family problems. Clinical examples are rich and detailed."

Marvin A. Acklin, PhD
Clinical Psychologist, Department of Psychiatry
University of Hawaii and Private Practice

"McCown and Johnson have merged current research with their clearly stated pragmatic approach to working with this most complex segment of the client population. This book offers clinicians clear guidelines for evaluation and brief intervention strategies for families in crisis. . . . An outstanding book that is direct, inclusive, focused, marvelously readable, and a useful resource of much-needed information for any therapist working with crisis-prone families."

Linda Chamberlain, PsyD
Psychologist
Psychological Resource Organization, Denver

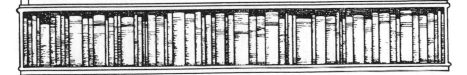

"An important and practical book for anyone working with treatment resistant families in any setting. . . . One of the few works that suggest pragmatic techniques for laying the foundation for future family therapy of medical inpatients."

Judith Holmes, PhD
Director of Neuropsychology
Lutheran General Hospital, Park Ridge, Illinois

"Must reading! A concise review of theory accompanied by excellent applications and case illustrations. . . . This book should go far to dispel the myth that treatment resistant families are hopeless."

Harry Galina, PhD
Center for Advanced Learning
Montreal

NOTES FOR PROFESSIONAL LIBRARIANS AND LIBRARY USERS

This is an original book title published by The Haworth Press, Inc. Unless otherwise noted in specific chapters with attribution, materials in this book have not been previously published elsewhere in any format or language.

CONSERVATION AND PRESERVATION NOTES

All books published by The Haworth Press, Inc. are printed on certified ph neutral, acid free book grade paper. This conforms to recommendations ensuring a book's long life without deterioration.

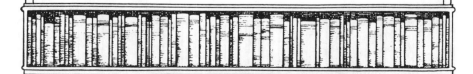

Therapy
with Treatment
Resistant Families
A Consultation-Crisis
Intervention Model

HAWORTH Marriage & the Family
Terry S. Trepper, PhD
Senior Editor

Therapy
with Treatment
Resistant Families
A Consultation-Crisis
Intervention Model

William George McCown, PhD
Judith Johnson, PhD
and Associates

The Haworth Press
New York • London • Norwood (Australia)

The Haworth Press, Inc., 10 Alice Street, Binghamton, NY 13904-1580 USA.

Library of Congress Cataloging-in-Publication Data

Therapy with treatment resistant families : a consultation-crisis intervention model / (edited by) William George McCown, Judith Johnson.
    p.   cm.
Includes bibliographical references and index.
ISBN 1-56024-244-2 (acid free paper).
1. Family psychotherapy. 2. Problem families–Counseling of. 3. Crisis intervention (Psychiatry) I. McCown, William George. II. Johnson, Judith, 1955– .
RC488.5.T492   1992
616.89´156–dc20

91-35618
CIP

This book is dedicated
to our families and students.

ABOUT THE AUTHORS

William George McCown, PhD, is Associate Professor of Mental Health Sciences at Hahnemann University and Medical School in Philadelphia. Dr. McCown has a broad area of research and clinical interests and has published over 50 professional papers.

Judith Johnson, PhD, is Director of Psychology at the Bucks/Upper Montgomery County Neurologic Group in North Wales, Pennsylvania, and Assistant Professor in the Department of Psychology at Villanova University. She is a family therapist and trained neuropsychologist and has extensive background in family-oriented crisis intervention. Dr. Johnson's principal area of clinical interest is in the use of family therapy with medical patients.

CONTENTS

Contributors and Associates

Chapter Two

Linda Frank, PhD, RNC
Barbara O'Toole, MDiv
Peter Koeppl, MA
John Beetar
Hahnemann University

Chapter Three

Aileen Fink, MA
Sharon Moore
Kimmy Kees
Hahnemann University

Chapter Four

Jody Talbott
Grand Rapids, Michigan

Tracy Neal
Rand Coleman
Hahnemann University

Chapter Five

Greg Stolcis, ACSW, LCSW
*Commonwealth of Virginia,
Office of Mental Health, Mental Retardation,
and Substance Abuse
Richmond, VA*

Chapter Six

Jan Vick, MSW ACSW
Metairie, LA

Chapter Seven

Deni Carise
Hahnemann University

Chapter Eight

Houman Verzandeh, PsyD
Philadelphia, PA

Chapter Nine

Steven Anderer
Adam Rosen
Hahnemann University and Villanova University School of Law

Chapter Ten

Lowell Birkett
Hahnemann University and Villanova University School of Law

Chapter Eleven

Daniel L. Skubick, MD
Neurologic Group of Bucks and Montgomery Counties, North Wales, PA

Preface

The problem that this book addresses is quite narrow: How should the clinician intervene with people from crisis-prone families who are unlikely to follow through with subsequent treatment? This is not a trivial issue. As many as one-third of families that the typical family-oriented clinician treats may fit this description.

Our attempts to answer this question go back a number of years. During the late 1970s, several of us, most of whom were at the time front line clinicians or paraprofessionals, became interested in how we could better help people from multi-problem families. We observed, as did numerous practitioners before us, that many of these multi-problem families were also crisis-prone. More specifically, two or three members in each of these families seemed to take turns experiencing psychiatric difficulties. Other family members often appeared to conspire against any outside helper trying to break this cycle.

Following many frustrating hours of clinical work, we began to hypothesize ways to intervene with these difficult clients. Although none of us were committed "systems" therapists at this time, the necessity of treating the entire family soon became apparent. During the early 1980s we became more involved in family-oriented crisis intervention. We collected data and communicated with other practitioners willing to do so. We also began exchanging techniques and notes with clinicians whose job it was to intervene with treatment resistant family systems. We experimented further–and made many mistakes. A few years later we were able to refine some of these techniques and test their underlying theory. Gradually, we began to see that the only way of successfully treating these high risk families–as we now called them–was to empower them to heal themselves, in their own manner and time.

This volume summarizes our clinical efforts to better understand a specific type of troublesome client family. It is neither a comprehensive guide to family therapy nor to crisis intervention. Many excellent texts exist in these areas. (However, to facilitate an understanding of family therapy theory and practice, Chapter Two offers a review of historic and contemporary trends in family therapy.) Furthermore, there are very few new ideas in this book. The family therapy techniques that we advance are a mixture of the variety of contemporary approaches to family therapy.

Nor is this a research volume. Most of our research on crisis-prone and treatment resistant families is presented elsewhere. The empirically-oriented clinician may experience some frustration with this, but this was a necessary compromise for a book aimed primarily at practitioners. Our research group continues to be active, and a separate empirical volume is planned for later.

Each of the chapters have several co-authors, many of whom are seasoned practitioners. Their participation is a strength of this volume. Other contributors are our present or former students, without whose input and help our ideas would have remained unwritten.

Special thanks are due to a number of people who made this book possible. They include Terry Trepper, PhD, Editor of the Haworth Series on Family Therapy. Pamela O'Connell and Eric Roland, Editorial Assistants at Haworth, showed extraordinary patience in the face of the first authors' chronic procrastination. Editorial assistance was provided by Lisa Hotovy and Jennifer Posa, without whose perseverance this book would still remain on a hard drive.

W.G.Mc.
Hahnemann University

J.L.J.
Villanova University

Chapter One

The Treatment Resistant Family

THE CONCEPT OF RESISTANCE

The phrase *treatment resistance* is an ambiguous term with varying meanings dependent upon the professional discipline and context of treatment. For example, in the practice of medicine resistance often refers to the probability a given treatment or course of therapeutic intervention will fail. In this context, a new strain of tuberculosis or virus may be resistant to traditional antibiotics, and the probability of success with commonly employed interventions is small. The problem of resistance in medicine is often lessened through accurate diagnosis of the disease or syndrome and application of the most appropriate treatment. If one treatment is ineffective, another is tried until a solution is found or until all options are exhausted.

In contrast, treatment resistance in psychotherapy is less precise and perhaps more complex than that found in medicine (Phillips, 1988). On one extreme, some schools of individual therapy deny that resistance even exists. Examples of this perspective are found in the writings of many existential and humanistic theorists, exemplified by writers such as Tormey (1985) who regards the patient's difficulties as a choice rather than an illness. Within such perspectives, therapy is actually a form of conversion whereby the patient is convinced that he or she is responsible for any difficulty and can exercise choices to effect change. Resistance to the therapist's interventions is simply one manifestation of the free will of the client.

On the other extreme, some schools of therapy view treatment resistance as a pervasive phenomena, influencing most clinical interaction. In classic psychoanalytic literature, resistance is conceptualized as any patient behavior that interrupts the progress of therapy. In this context, missed appointments, late arrivals, or un-

1

productive therapy sessions are viewed as indicators of resistance to the analytic work (Cameron & Rychlak, 1985). The analytic patient who is strongly resistant may remain in therapy for years, with little demonstrated insight or behavioral change. In these situations patients are often admonished to work harder and continue their present course of treatment (Brown, 1940).

Unlike medicine, treatment resistance in individual therapy is often associated with an attribution of responsibility on the part of the patient. For example, psychoanalytic or neoanalytic therapies commonly include the patient as a party to the therapeutic failure. It is also common to interpret resistance as a failure on the part of the therapist to effectively manage countertransference issues. In contrast, cognitive and behavioral individual therapies often place responsibility for resistance squarely on the therapist. Treatment resistance is usually attributed to technical difficulties involving therapeutic competence, experience, or technique. If a patient has been unable to extinguish a phobia or correct cognitive distortions, the therapist's skills or technical competence may be implicated.

Treatment resistance in family therapy is probably more complex than in individual therapy (Coleman, 1985). It certainly is believed to be more common inasmuch as most schools of family therapy anticipate it, at least to some extent (e.g., Ackerman, 1958; Haley, 1976; Keeney, 1982; Minuchin, 1974; Stanton, 1980; Stanton & Todd, 1982; Stuart, 1980). Compared to individual therapy, there is usually at least one person in the family system who is uncooperative with the therapist's and perhaps other family members' treatment goals. A husband may insist on marital therapy, while his wife insists that "Nothing is wrong." Or a single parent may bring in a brood of rebellious children, who jointly maintain that "Mom is the crazy one, not us." This contrasts with individual therapy where it is relatively rare to treat someone who is overtly unmotivated for treatment.

Writers addressing resistance in family therapy have often tended to fault the therapist for family therapy failures (e.g., Haley, 1980). When the family abruptly terminates treatment or fails to comply with the therapist's recommendations, it is often assumed the therapist was inexperienced, careless, or in error (Fisch, Weakland, & Segal, 1983). Failures in family therapy may also be attributed to the supervisor or to the notion that the provider of therapy has unresolved family problems (Bowen, 1978). Lack of training and ethnic or racial insensitivity are also commonly invoked as explanations of treatment resistance or failure. Finally, lack of treatment success may be attributed to the "system," social forces, or other broadly defined factors (Geismer & La Sorte, 1964).

It is rarely acknowledged that different families may require individually tailored types of intervention to overcome resistance (Kaplan, 1984). Although many agree in principle that careful initial assessment of the family is important, there is little evidence that clinicians systematically modify treatment interventions based upon an initial evaluation of the likelihood of resistance. The major purpose of this volume is to illustrate that resistant families can be initially identified and ensuing treatment can be specifically adjusted to ensure maximal effectiveness. Practical intervention with treatment resistant families does not fault the therapist or the family for failure. Instead, it targets specific aspects of family systems functioning and family behavior in an attempt to further the goal of treatment compliance (Kaplan, 1986). Although not a "medical model" of treatment, the strategy we advocate with resistant families involves careful evaluation and diagnosis of a family's problems, based on past history and indicators of treatment resistance.

VARIETIES OF FAMILY TREATMENT RESISTANCE

A discussion of ways to overcome family resistance should begin by defining the phrase. Not surprisingly, the term "treatment resistant family" has a variety of meanings, depending upon which treatment phase or component the family resists (Lombardi, 1990). Below, we identify several major forms of resistance. There are certainly more. Anderson and Stewart (1983) identify more than 40 sources of resistance in family therapy. Although our discussion is not exhaustive, it is indicative of major ways families can be viewed as treatment resistant with subsequent interference in maximum therapeutic progress.

Resistance can be used to describe either the unsuccessful results of family therapy or as a description of difficulties involved in the interactive therapeutic process. To borrow the technical language from psychotherapy outcome research, resistance is both an outcome and process variable. Regarding outcome, families that fail in therapy are often labeled resistant, especially by therapists treating them. Such labeling provides a convenient explanation, if not excuse for why the family did not improve. However, viewing failure as "resistance" may often be done to preserve the therapist's or supervisor's ego (Kottler & Blau, 1989).

Families may also be labeled as resistant on the basis of demographic factors. Coleman (1985) notes that socioeconomic and cultural variables may affect the course of family therapy. Indeed, low income or disadvantaged families are often labeled as treatment resistant (Schlesinger, 1963). This label is based on the fact that these families are often believed to have a poor prognosis in therapy, at least as it is practiced by many therapists. Often, however, the therapist's cultural, racial and ethnic insensitivities are at least equal in importance to family characteristics in treatment resistance (Tseng & Hsu, 1991).

Outcome labeling need not be limited to retrospective accounts. Upon initial treatment contact a family may be labeled as resistant if they are *exceptionally pathological and unlikely to change*. For example, a family where incest is practiced may be likely to continue this behavior despite extraordinary treatment efforts. Similarly, an alcoholic family may be at great risk to continue their collective dysfunctional patterns (Kaufman, 1985). In these cases the label of resistance is an indication of the probability that certain families are not likely to benefit from therapeutic efforts, even if they do participate in treatment. When services are rationed, as they often are in the public sector, therapists informally allocate precious therapy time in part by determining the family's resistance to change. This is perhaps the closest to the medical definition of resistance. The principal guiding the intervention is substantially the same as medical triaging in a busy emergency room in that services should be administered to those most likely to benefit.

Another type of outcome resistance is associated with *deterioration of one or more family members while in treatment* (Ackerman, 1961). Based upon the belief the family is a system of interacting components, improvement in one area of systemic functioning or in one family member may be met with deterioration of functioning in another area or family member. An example is often encountered in the alcoholic family, where a parent's drinking ceases, but the children become more symptomatic (Steinglass, 1977). The net positive therapeutic gain in terms of the total system's well-being is little to nothing.

We do not know how frequently this type of resistance occurs. The deterioration rate for marital and family therapy for one or more members in the system has been estimated at 5 to 10 percent (Gurman & Kniskern, 1978). This figure is comparable to that of clients receiving a broad range of individual psychotherapies (Bergin, 1967; Lambert, Bergin & Collins, 1977), and suggests family therapy may be no more risky than individual treatment. However, the dearth of existent studies suggests that therapists be aware that family therapy has the potential for being harmful as well as beneficial.

In the next few chapters we will argue that specific types of families are very likely to deteriorate following initial family intervention. This is because they have a propensity to terminate treatment early. Many popular family therapy interventions act by increasing stress to the family system or by destabilizing a pathological but stable family hierarchy. These interventions-which may be spectacularly helpful with families who remain in therapy-may be harmful if the family abruptly quits treatment. The goal of the therapist is to identify these families before treatment starts.

Treatment resistance to the process of therapy is demonstrated when families fail to comply with *initial recommendations for treatment*. In other words, resistance can precede initial contact with the therapist. For example, a family may present in crisis to a family physician or emergency room and receive a referral for ongoing treatment. They may subsequently "lose" or "forget" the referral, or simply claim to be too busy to pursue mental health treatment. A typical pattern for these families is for one or more members to present to a local agency in a state of psychiatric emergency, where elaborate plans are formulated for treatment intervention. However, the family frequently disappears as soon as the initial crisis is over. All too often, the crisis repeats itself sometime in the future.

A second type of treatment process resistance involves systems that demonstrate *superficial cooperation*, but surreptitiously act to mitigate effective treatment. Despite frequent emotional distress, these families frustrate the best intentions of therapists they encounter. The methods these families have of effectively sabotaging therapy are varied and occasionally ingenious. More frequently, however, they are as mundane as simply claiming to lack the time or the money for additional therapy at precisely the point where real change is demanded. Fisch, Weakland, and Segal (1983) label these families as "window shoppers," a clever phrase implying their true lack of commitment to change. The Family Study below illustrates a "window shopping" family.

Family Study 1.1. The Ellerby Family

> Pat Ellerby, 34, and her husband John, 36, were well known to every mental health professional in a tri-county area. Pat and John have an extensive history of domestic violence and crisis service utilization. Together, they had made 11 calls to the crisis intervention service of their county mental health center during the two past years. Pat has also been sheltered three times at the local women's shelter. John has been expelled from home by his wife at least twice as often and spent many nights sleeping in his car. The couple is also well known to the local police.
>
> Following each incident of domestic violence, the couple repeats a familiar pattern. After a few days they joyfully reunite and vow to change their behaviors. They then seek treatment at a nearby community agency. Initially, the couple appears positive and compliant. However, at the point where the therapist requires real change from the family, Pat and John find an excuse to terminate treatment. Within a few weeks there is another incident of domestic violence and another call to the crisis service. The cycle simply repeats.

Another type of process resistance occurs when families attempt to *dictate the terms of treatment to the therapist.* Fisch, Weakland, and Segal (1983) label this family as the "restrictive" type and note they are commonly found in family therapy clinics. The resistance is usually first revealed in an initial struggle over who should be seen for treatment. Family members will often insist that particular members be included or excluded from treatment. When the therapist does not abide by these wishes, the family may refuse to cooperate and subsequently terminate treatment.

Equally resistant is the family that goes to excessive effort to "therapist shop." There is an apparent irony in this, since treatment resistant families are more likely than non-resistant families to prematurely terminate regardless of therapist characteristics. Yet precisely because they are so disagreeable, they go to elaborate lengths to find particular therapists or modalities that suit them best, at least for the time being (Levy & McCown, 1983). Often, though only when their entire history is known, families that are resistant to treatment may resemble "therapy addicts." This seeming paradox of resistant families simultaneously sabotaging treatment and excessively using treatment involves an underlying theme surrounding the issue of control. That is, these families simply desire treatment on their own terms, and are wary of interventions over which they do not have complete control. The Family Study below illustrates this tendency to be both "under-" and "over-utilizers" of mental health services.

Family Study 1.2. The Charters Family

Bob and Teddy Charters were an upper middle-class family. Ted was a respected, if hotheaded chemist, whose brilliance in his career was overshadowed by his inability to get along with coworkers. He had been treated in private psychoanalysis three times a week for five years. He also saw a pastoral counselor for therapy once a week for the past year. Teddy, a social worker, was diagnosed by her general practitioner as being depressed. She was then placed in private group and individual therapy on a weekly basis, also covered by insurance. The couple had also been in marital therapy for four years, paid out of pocket. Three of the four children were in private individual psychodynamically-oriented therapy. When the family was in one of their frequent crises, the mother and father had a list of seven therapists to call.

Because of the truant behavior of two of the children, a

school counselor strongly recommended family therapy in addition to the therapeutic regimen that was already in place. The family dutifully contacted an appropriate therapist and voiced an initial enthusiasm about at long last finding some "real help" for their children. However, after two sessions, the parents stated that they wished to discontinue treatment because it was not helpful. The therapist urged them to stay, promising eventual results. The parents tentatively agreed.

After three more sessions, the parents stated that, although helpful, treatment was too expensive. Fees were reduced to make the treatment more affordable. Two sessions later the couple stated that they would have to terminate family treatment because the time was inconvenient. Somewhat exasperated, the therapist adjusted the time to the family's liking. The next session the family announced that they would have to terminate because the family was "too tired with all this extra therapy."

Teddy called the therapist a month later in extreme distress. She explained that her oldest son had been expelled from school for truancy and she wished to resume family treatment immediately. The therapist was dumbfounded at the family's change of attitude. This time, however, Teddy made it clear that her husband and other children would not be involved in the process. "I think family therapy ought to include just the two of us. You do agree, don't you?"

Families also demonstrate process resistance if they are consciously or unconsciously *manipulative or otherwise "difficult"* (Fisch, Weakland, & Segal, 1983). Often, these families may exhaust a particular agency's resources and then quickly advance to the next available treatment facility. The resistant family may facilitate its transition to another agency by complaining about their previous therapist. For example, they may denigrate previous treatment providers or disparage the facilities.

Difficult families may also be proficient at appealing to therapists' egotism by providing glowing comments regarding the therapist's clinical acumen or intervention skills. The therapist who treats resistant families frequently hears that he or she was chosen by the client family because of special abilities that are known throughout the community. The family may further appeal to the therapist's sense of competency by stating that the reason for their history of frequent treatment failure was due to a lack of skill on the part of numerous past practitioners.

Furthermore, difficult families may deliberately or inadvertently become adept at exploiting rifts between individually-oriented and family-oriented therapists. Both groups of therapists may fall prey to the complaints by members of a treatment resistant family that "The other therapist (that works in a different modality) just doesn't help me like your approach does." Family therapists who are sensitive to their professional status among other practitioners may seem particularly vulnerable to this tactic.

Process resistance is often manifest in the desire of the family to "fix" their "disturbed" member or members. This phenomena is well known to family therapists and has been labeled by Ackerman (1967) as "family scapegoating." In scapegoating, the family targets one or more members as the sole source of their dysfunction. Families believe that if this member could simply be "healed," the family would return to its previously harmonious state. Often these families attempt to "dump" the dysfunctional family members into whatever mental health system they can find.

When the therapist working with the resistant family refuses to accept the belief that the family's problem does not extend beyond that of one or two targeted members, the family will typically react with anger towards the therapist. When this occurs, the family often terminates treatment with both the family and the therapist feeling misunderstood, ineffectual, or even indignant (Cade, 1975).

Another form of process resistance similar to scapegoating occurs when the family *mistakenly attributes its level of dysfunction to a single environmental event* or to circumstances that cannot be changed. For example, a family might believe the dysfunctional behavior of a schizophrenic son to be related to drug use on a distant occasion. In another instance, one family we recently worked with believed the father's incestuous behavior was due to the fact he had contracted malaria while in World War II. Usually, the purported causal event contributing to family dysfunction occurred in the distant past and is unchangeable. The event may also assume mythological status in the family's legacy (Framo, 1982). Therapists who reject outright the role of this past event often find that they cannot work with these families.

A variant of this form of resistance occurs when the family ascribes its dysfunctional behavior *solely* to genetics or "chemical imbalances." One example we recently encountered was a grandmother who excused the criminal behavior of her drug addicted grandson by saying that he is "a good boy, but just has some bad blood." The implications are that his behavior is outside of the family's control. Similarly, some self-help groups for parents of children with major psychiatric disorders have been critical of family theorists' interventions. Some insist that schizophrenia and other major psychopathologies should be treated exclusively from a biological perspective, and thus are resistant to the idea family dynamics may play a role in maintaining dysfunctional patterns.

Most family therapists recognize the influence of genetics and neurobiological factors on behavior (L'Abate, Farrar, & Serritella, 1992). Substantial evidence exists that many psychiatric disorders have a genetic component, which in some cases may be quite large. Moreover, therapists almost universally recognize that pharmacological therapy is often indicated for a variety of psychiatric disorders. However, family processes are a better predictor of current family members' symptomatology and symptom intensity than individual psychiatric diagnoses. The prognosis of persons with major psychiatric disorders depends largely on their environment, of which the family system is perhaps the most important component. We will return to this point later in the chapter.

THE IMPACT OF RESISTANCE

Despite the variety of resistances a family may manifest, the overall impact on the therapist and on therapy is similar. Extreme resistance, either in degree or frequency, foments disillusionment and hostility on the part of the therapist (Anderson & Stewart, 1983). Hopelessness and insecurity may then develop, which may be especially difficult for the novice therapist to manage (Lombardi, 1990). In our experience, therapists who abandon a systems modality usually do so in frustration following repeated experience with very resistant or difficult families. These practitioners often complain to their more family-oriented colleagues that "Family therapy just didn't work for me."

Treatment resistance, regardless of cause or variety, is also associated with a higher likelihood that therapeutic interventions will fail. This is true for both outcome and process resistance. The treatment resistant family does not work as "hard" or as "well" in therapy as the non-resistant family (Levy & McCown, 1983). Essentially, they are less conscientious regarding therapy and therefore less likely to actually perform behaviors that the therapist suggests or orchestrates. Evidence for this is provided by McCown and Johnson (1992c), who found significant negative correlations between a number of indices of family resistance and therapist ratings of positive outcome in family therapy. These include missed sessions, lateness, failure to implement previously agreed-upon tasks, attending therapy under the influence of substances, and spontaneous termination of treatment by individual family members while the rest of the family remains in treatment. Families with high levels of resistance were also found to be more likely to call the therapist between sessions, avoid paying fees, and withhold informed consent to contact other family members. Finally, resistant families were more likely to seek treatment from two or more therapy agencies simultaneously.

EARLY THERAPY TERMINATION: THE MOST EXTREME PROCESS RESISTANCE

Meichenbaum and Turk (1987) have discussed techniques for coping with therapeutic "nonadherence" in individual therapy. Their excellent volume contains many useful strategies for coping with family resistance as well. For example, they advocate that it is incumbent upon the therapist to anticipate, expect, and predict resistance to change. They recommend a number of strategies to minimize nonadherence, including customizing treatment, involving the family, and mobilizing community supports. Perhaps most importantly for our present discussion, they note that nonadherent clients are likely to terminate therapy early, against the recommendations of the therapist. Clearly, the most effective and dramatic form of resistance is either to quit therapy or avoid beginning it at all.

The notion of termination as the most severe type of resistance is not new. Its lineage can be traced to the Freudian tradition which assumes the principal of psychic determinism: everything patients do in therapy has meaning and purpose (Freud, 1938). Patients who are late for appointments are less resistant than those who sporadically miss therapy sessions. These latter patients are less resistant than those who terminate during the middle point of the analytic process. The most resistant are those who do not have the ego strength to begin or sustain therapy beyond the first few sessions (Brown, 1940).

In recent years researchers have suggested the use of brief therapies to overcome the deficits inherent in early termination of treatment (Phillips, 1988). Crisis intervention theory (discussed in Chapter Four) was developed, in part, to reach clients that were less likely to comply with traditional interventions and more likely to terminate treatment after only a few sessions. Writers such as Bloom (1981) argued that the first session in individual psychotherapy is often the last. Accordingly, he developed an effective one-session treatment for individual therapy clients who are unlikely to return for further treatment. Other forms of brief therapies are rapidly gaining in popularity, in part to minimize client resistance but also because of high costs associated with more traditional and lengthy interventions (Phares, 1992).

Termination or avoidance of treatment as a form of resistance is of little consequence in family therapy if it is rarely encountered. Estimates of the prevalence of this type of resistance are difficult to obtain, inasmuch as it is usually impossible to gather data on individuals who have left treatment. An exception is when families are mandated into treatment by the judicial process, such as when probation officers suggest or require family therapy. Even in this situation where the family has strong legal incentives to seek treatment, family compliance rates-making and keeping an initial appointment with a family therapist-are often no more than 25 percent (McCown & Johnson, 1985). Undoubtedly, noncompliance rates are much higher when the referral is made by non-judicial agents such as school psychologists, physicians, ministers, or social service agencies.

Both rates of initial family therapy "no shows" and premature termination from treatment are easier to ascertain, since they can be obtained from clinical records. Undoubtedly, incidence rates of these forms of resistance vary widely, and depend upon on a number of interacting factors. These include the types of families being served, the therapy setting, orientation of the treatment provider, economic status, and perhaps even the time of year. However, such data may be extremely important for practitioners, inasmuch as it can help them target treatment more appropriately. Surprisingly, there are few studies that examine the rates of these extreme forms of treatment resistance in family therapy.

McCown and Johnson (1991) examined the frequency of early termination and initial session "no shows" at three family-oriented clinics. These included a family therapy agency in the Southeast, a Midwestern mental health center, and a family clinic connected with a major Southern medical center. Sixteen percent of families failed to attend their first session (excluding those who postponed their sessions). Among families without judicial involvement, this initial no show rate was slightly over 21 percent. Furthermore, another 25 percent of families terminated treatment by the third session. In other words, more than two out of five families who initially requested family therapy failed to receive more than three sessions.

These authors also found a highly significant correlation of $(r = -.32)$ between the previous number of early terminations from therapy and the number of sessions the client family received in their most recent therapy endeavor. The greater the number of previous treatment failures, the fewer the number of sessions families were likely to attend. (A correlation of this magnitude is more remarkable inasmuch as it was attenuated by a restriction in range of both the independent and dependent variables.) The authors also ascertained the modal and mean numbers of therapy sessions families with a previous history of treatment noncompliance will experience during their newest treatment efforts before they terminate. For families with a history of four or more early terminations-16 percent of the families studied-the modal number of sessions actually attended was three, with a mean of 3.8.

Although this study has limitations and requires replication, some conclusions warrant attention. These findings suggest that families with a history of early termination are likely to repeat this pattern in present treatment efforts. Therapists must realize that families with a history of treatment failure will probably not remain in treatment. Ideally, interventions designed to assist such families should be geared towards quick completion, probably in one to three sessions. Treatment plans that disregard this imperative are unrealistic and likely to be ineffective.

Why do families drop out of treatment? This is a complex question, indeed. Certain disorders, such as substance abuse or other addictive behaviors have often been associated with treatment resistance, including early termination (L'Abate, Farrar, & Serritella, 1992; McCown & Johnson, 1992b). Other specific characteristics of family systems, such as the closed system (discussed in Chapter Two), have also been implicated (Satir, 1967). Later chapters will further discuss hypothesized explanations of extreme family resistance. It is unlikely that any one explanation is sufficient, and there may be as many reasons for resistance as there are families being treated.

An understanding of the implications of treatment resistance for family therapy may be more important than precise etiology. As discussed above, the resistant family will exert less effort and be less successful in family therapy (Anderson & Stewart, 1983). When resistance is mild or moderate, a number of techniques can be used to overcome the family's reluctance to change. Interventions such as paradoxes (L'Abate, 1986), reframing (Fisch, Weakland, & Segal, 1983), symptom prescription (Haley, 1976), and induction of family crises can be effective as long as families remain in treatment. Structural and strategic therapists (discussed in Chapter Two) have been particularly clever in developing techniques to overcome mild or moderate resistance (e.g., Stanton & Todd, 1981). However, these interventions and many others commonly practiced by family therapists will not work if the family practices the most intense form of resistance, namely early termination. Extremely resistant families-those with a history of multiple early termination from treatment-are likely to repeat this pattern. Traditional family therapy interventions may be ineffective with this group because they do not remain in treatment long enough to benefit.

A corollary implication is that extremely resistant families are at greater risk of deteriorating in family therapy. Along these lines, McCown and Johnson (1992c) found that families with a history of treatment failure were more likely to show a deterioration in functioning following family intervention. This likely occurs because family therapy interventions often destabilize the family system, at least initially (O'Shee & Jessee, 1982). As later chapters indicate, many family therapy interventions are tantamount to invasive surgery on the family system. For maximal efficacy, a therapist often needs to be influential, in control, and occasionally disruptive of the family system (Gurman & Kniskern, 1978). Families that experience initial destabilization who terminate before they can reorganize are never allowed the opportunity to heal from this disruption.

Therapists working with potentially resistant families face a dilemma. Interventions must effectively challenge the family to implement genuine modification or change. Otherwise, such interventions merely provide a temporary solution to a dysfunctional system, changing nothing in the process. On the other hand, therapy must proceed with great caution. The challenge with family intervention within the treatment resistant system is to provide the impetus for further treatment without damaging the family should it abruptly discontinue therapy, a very real possibility. This procedure is both an art and a science and is a major emphasis of this volume.

TREATMENT RESISTANCE AND FAMILY CRISES

The crux of our approach with resistant families is that an understanding of the dynamics of family crises and crisis intervention is vital. There are a number of reasons for this. One is that the treatment resistant family usually enters treatment only following a significant family disruption or crisis. This was demonstrated in a study by McCown and Johnson (1992c), who examined archival records of 187 families. Treatment resistance was determined by several variables including past history of early termination, therapist ratings, and frequency counts of noncompliant activities, such as arriving late or excluding key family members from treatment. Each of these variables correlated moderately with each other. A factor analysis was used to construct a "resistance index" of therapy variables, with higher scores being associated with greater resistance. Families with resistance index scores above the median were operationally defined as resistant families and were compared to those scoring below the median.

Resistant families were significantly more likely to have presented for treatment following a crisis. Furthermore, there was a moderate correlation (.38) between the therapists' ratings of the precipitating crisis and resistance scores. Resistant families had a higher "threshold" of what constituted a family crisis warranting treatment. Moreover, resistant families had a much higher level of daily family stress prior to treatment entry than nonresistant families. Resistant families were also significantly more likely to be forced into treatment following contact with community agencies, such as a school psychologist, the court, or a social service agency. Finally, resistant families had a much longer period of having experienced the presenting problem prior to seeking treatment than nonresistant families.

An understanding of crisis intervention is also necessary because treatment resistant families have a high comorbidity, or coincidence, of crisis-proneness (McCown & Johnson, 1991, 1992a). Later chapters will address potential explanations for this overlap between crisis-proneness and treatment resistance. For purposes of the present discussion, it is more important to address the frequency with which such client families are encountered.

Unfortunately, this issue is presently difficult to clarify due to a paucity of empirical data. Reviews of the literature on individual patients who are psychiatric emergency "repeaters" (not families) have been presented by Nurius (1983; 1984) and Ellison, Blum, and Barsky (1986). Repeaters are patients that are both treatment resistant and crisis-prone, as indicated by use of an emergency room rather than a therapist and frequency of emergency room visits. Barker (1990) notes that these types of patients are relatively common. In fact, Ellison et al. (1986) found that between 7 percent and 18 percent of psychiatric emergency service patients are repeaters. Furthermore, repeaters were found to account for up to one-third of the total emergency room psychiatric visits.

Data collection regarding treatment resistance and crisis-proneness in *families* is considerably more difficult to obtain than for individuals. There are a number of reasons for this. First, facilities involved primarily with individuals (such as emergency rooms or most mental health centers) rarely obtain or maintain detailed data on the crises of significant family members. Secondly, when such data is obtained it may be distorted or inaccurate. Third, many mental health agencies impose some form of treatment rationing regarding crisis services which may act to limit access of these families to treatment. For example, many health maintenance organizations severely limit the number of emergency contacts client families can make.

Only one study has examined this co-occurrence in families. McCown and Johnson (1992c) examined archival records across several intervention sites which treated psychiatric emergencies. Crisis repeaters accounted for approximately 35 percent of all emergency patient contacts. Of these repeaters, about 74 percent had a history of noncompliance with treatment, as indicated by failure to follow recommendations from the previous intervention. Of this group, 54 percent had family members that also had a history of an episode of psychiatric crisis. Therefore, about 14 percent of all individuals receiving mental health services (one in seven) were from a family system that was both crisis-prone and treatment resistant.

McCown and Johnson (1991; 1992c) have labeled families that are both treatment resistant and crisis-prone as "high risk family systems." This name is based on the fact that such families are at high risk to both sabotage treatment and subsequently experience additional crises. They are also at high risk to exhaust the efforts and good intentions of care providers. Finally, they are at high risk to experience eventual and severe deterioration of functioning in multiple areas (McCown & Johnson, 1991), including histories of substance abuse, incest, child abuse, and major psychopathology.

Data from McCown and Johnson (1991) suggests that these "high risk" families place large demands on their service providers. These authors found that high risk families, those families with a prior history of crisis-proneness and treatment resistance, require almost twice as many staff hours for each crisis than do other less pathological families. Furthermore, these families were found to be five times as likely to discontinue treatment against their therapist's advice as families without such histories.

Although crisis-proneness, treatment resistance, and high risk frequently overlap, the terms are not synonymous. As Figure 1.1 indicates, families can be crisis-prone or treatment resistant without having the two characteristics in combination. However, the interaction between crisis-proneness and treatment resistance in family systems is so common and pronounced that it warrants its own term. Throughout this volume we will use the phrase "high risk family" to describe family systems displaying the pattern of a history of repeated crises with subsequent resistance to therapeutic intervention.

SYSTEMS INTERVENTION WITH HIGHLY RESISTANT FAMILIES

During the last decade we began to investigate characteristics of the resistant and crisis-prone client. Initially, we attempted to ex-

FIGURE 1.1. Crisis-Proneness and Treatment Resistance

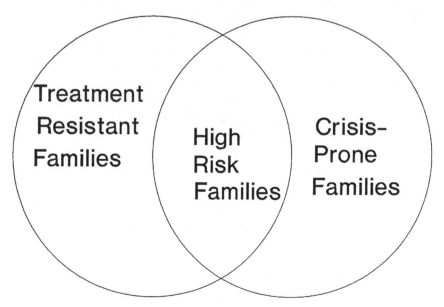

plain and predict patient recidivism and treatment resistance from an individual perspective. That is, we tried to demonstrate specific patient characteristics as primary determinants of both crisis-proneness and treatment resistance. Ultimately, we realized the importance of family systemic variables in regulating the behavior of crisis recidivists.

This is not to minimize the importance of individual differences and diagnostic categories in treatment compliance and therapeutic efficacy. A wealth of behavioral science literature has examined individual factors associated with positive therapeutic outcome. Often, such information is invaluable for the clinician. For example, such factors as conscientiousness, intelligence, impulsivity, openness, tolerance for ambiguity, and agreeableness are related to positive outcomes and compliance in psychiatric treatment (Phares, 1992). Similarly, diagnostic classifications possess important predictive and explanatory value regarding treatment compliance and crisis-proneness. Substance abuse disorders, the schizophrenias and some personality disorders are often associated with poor treatment compliance and frequent crises. In contrast, diagnoses such as phobias, adjustment disorders, and depression are less likely to involve a cycle of treatment rejection and subsequent crisis.

However, explanations solely emphasizing individually-oriented etiologies of the cycle of crisis-proneness and resistance are not sufficient inasmuch as they are incapable of explaining why and when such clients experience crises. One of the least understood aspects of the client who "recycles" is the answer to the query of "Why now?" Unless additional factors are considered outside of the individual, the process of crisis timing will appear to be essentially random. Clinicians who confine themselves to examining individually-oriented personality and diagnostic variables regarding crisis-proneness will remain stymied in their understanding of these seeming "random events" (Chamberlain, 1991). Our contention is that specific techniques tailored to highly resistant family systems may decrease family interference and maximize the likelihood the family will benefit from interventions.

The remaining chapters of this book will discuss theory and methods of treating families who are extremely treatment resistant, especially those who are crisis-prone or "high risk." Our emphasis is on what we consider the most serious manifestation of resistance, early termination of therapy by one or more family members. This includes both families that vacillate regarding their decision to seek initial intervention and families who make initial therapist contact, but fail to follow through with subsequent treatment. However, we feel our theory and clinical methods are appropriate for families with less severe forms of resistance as well.

We will propose a series of interventions designed to reduce treatment resistance and potential crisis-proneness while maximizing the desire of the system to overcome its dysfunction. Our strategy is to intervene first in the presenting crisis, defusing it sufficiently so that the family can function, but not so stringently that the family's motivation for treatment is dissipated. Following this, we advocate a change of therapeutic roles to that of a consultant, working with the family to avoid their propensity for early termination. Unlike many traditional family therapy interventions, the techniques we advocate empower families to change themselves, rather than mandate them to respond to systemic disruption. The power of the therapist in the family system is de-emphasized, with greater consideration placed upon allowing the family to change its own environment, and eventually, itself.

Before we discuss our specific sequence of interventions, we will have to take a few necessary detours. Many of the clinicians who perform therapy with extremely resistant systems do not have a background or credentialing in the field of family therapy. They are often social workers, counselors, probation officers, physicians, nurses, addictions workers, pastors, and psychologists who work with agencies that are individually oriented. Unfortunately, even 45 years after its inception, many practitioners are minimally exposed to the history and concepts of family therapy. Therefore, Chapter Two will provide a very brief historical introduction to family systems theory, as well as an overview of major "schools" of family therapy. The seasoned family therapist may wish to skim or ignore all but the last section, where we discuss recent developments in nonlinear and dynamical systems theory and their application to family therapy.

Chapter Three is primarily a general discussion of the literature regarding family stress, coping methods, and crises. Major theories of stress and family functioning will be reviewed briefly. We present data suggesting that treatment resistant, crisis-prone, and high risk families are different from other families in the way that stressors effect their systems. We then propose several general therapeutic interventions based upon these differences.

Chapter Four will discuss the history of and necessity for crisis intervention therapy with resistant families. As in Chapters Two and Three, our discussion is not meant to be an exhaustive discussion of crisis intervention theory and techniques. There are many excellent volumes regarding crisis intervention and even family-oriented crisis intervention. Most are more comprehensive than the present book, and certainly worth reading. This chapter has a much more restricted focus. We limit our discussion primarily to establishing the rationale of interventions for resistant families unlikely to continue in treatment past the initial crisis phase.

The remainder of this book will highlight clinical methods developed by our group and colleagues for treating resistant families. They may be families that refuse to realize the seriousness of their dysfunction. Or, in the case of high risk families, they are systems that despite histories of numerous difficulties, believe once the crisis has passed underlying difficulties are absolved and need for continued treatment is unnecessary. Hence, by their very nature, both groups of families may be seen for a very few number of sessions, and the majority of our interventions presented are designed to be performed within one to three therapy sessions. We admit immediately that our model is not universally applicable to all problems. In fact, the final chapters are firm caveats regarding the limitations of our approach.

Finally, we want to note that we presently have less empirical data to offer the practitioner than is our preference. Thus, much of our treatment application will rely upon case history illustrations. We anticipate that ongoing and future research can lend greater empirical credence to some of the assumptions and methods we have found to be useful and presently advocate with treatment resistant families. We would like nothing more than for the research community to improve upon our interventions and practice, further refining our techniques until they are obsolete and have been replaced by better methods of intervention.

Chapter Two

Families and Family Therapy:
A Brief History and Current Status

HISTORICAL CONCEPTS OF THE FAMILY
AND FAMILY THERAPY

Individual psychotherapy originated with the ancients, although it emerged as a profession only about a hundred or so years ago. There are numerous accounts in early literature of the precursors of modern psychotherapy. For example, the ancient Greek philosophers suggested that the emotionally troubled should seek the advice of wise elders. In the Pentateuch YHWH (the ancient Hebrew word for God) offered direct guidance to distraught Patriarchs. Perhaps a thousand years later, Galen, the Second Century physician, taught his students the curative value of listening to their patients' emotional problems, formulating a diagnosis, and then furnishing sound recommendations. Throughout the Middle Ages and into the modern era, it is obvious that much of the role played by contemporary psychotherapists was adeptly managed, perhaps more successfully than today, by the clergy (Frank, 1961).

Family therapy, unlike individual therapy, is unique in that there are few historic counterparts to it in ancient and pre-twentieth century literature. If we expected to find parallels of current family interventions recorded in ancient sacred or secular literature we would probably be disappointed. In the Old Testament, YHWH occasionally intervened in domestic matters, as in Genesis 16: 1-16 when He reproached Sar'ai's treatment of her pregnant handmaiden Hagar. However, most family disputes were settled by YHWH or El Shaeddai ("God, the one of the Mountains") directly and by divine fiat, usually by telling the husband what decision to make for his wife and children (e.g., Genesis 17: 15-21). In Genesis 18:9-16, YHWH avoids the chance to perform "couple's therapy" by refusing to communicate directly to Sarah, who is forced to listen separately to the voice of the LORD from behind Abraham's tent door.

This situation regarding family intervention is not much different in the New Testament. For an example, an Angel of the Lord speaks to Zechari'ah telling him that his elderly wife Elizabeth will soon find herself pregnant for the first time (Luke 1:8-23). Unfortunately, Zechari'ah is struck dumb for his disbelief and doesn't even get the opportunity to tell Elizabeth what will happen to her! The story of the Annunciation is more equitable to women, but not to the married couple. The Angel of the Lord informs Mary alone of the upcoming birth of Jesus (Luke 1:26-38). Joseph, an obviously important figure in this story, is told of this momentous family event at a later date and through a dream (Matthew 1:18-26).

It is probable that family therapy is a product of recent years because our conceptions of "family" is a modern one. This contrasts with the social institution of marriage, which is naturally older, and appears to be universal (Parsons & Bales, 1955). In Genesis 3:24 we read: "Therefore a man leaves his father and his mother and cleaves to his wife and they become one flesh" (Revised Standard Version). The immeasurable affinity between man and woman is illustrated in the statement that God made the woman from man's rib. It is what happens after marriage and especially after childbirth that is more likely to vary across cultures and epochs.

The word *family* came into the English language between the late fourteenth and early fifteenth centuries (Williams, 1976). Previously, there was no single term for the concept. The immediate forerunner of this term was the Latin word familia, meaning household. An alternative and perhaps antecedent etiology, familus, is Latin for servant. Thus, with introduction of the word family, there was a fusion of both close relationship and of servitude. Not surprisingly, men spoke of having families, while women spoke of having husbands and other kin.

During the fifteenth and sixteenth centuries the word family became more closely aligned to the notion of kin group, or even clan (Morganson, 1897). In the King James version of the Bible, family was restricted to words meaning "a wide kin group," often closer to our concept of "tribe" (Genesis 10:5; Jeremiah 31:1; Ezekiel 20:32). Relations between parent and children were usually translated as "near kin." By the end of the sixteenth century the term family was being used to describe persons of a common household, or those living under one roof, regardless of relatedness or cohesion. Servants were said to be "part of the family," not out of paternal benevolence, but simply because they were chattel that dwelled in close proximity to the master (Morganson, 1897).

Between the seventeenth and nineteenth centuries the current distinction between nuclear and extended families arose. A nuclear family is a kinship network limited to the husband, wife, and children, while an extended family includes other relatives, often of indirect lineage. It is difficult to trace the complex history of development of this distinction, which is by no means universal (Williams, 1976). Nor is it possible to agree upon a date for its emergence. However, the preeminence of the word family as referring primarily to a "small kin group" was probably not established among the population-at-large before the early nineteenth century.

The nuclear family arose in large part because of the demands for more efficient productivity. Many sociologists believe that the nuclear family was an economic unit necessary for the development of capitalism (Dahrendorf, 1967), which occurred with the rise of wage labor among the middle- and lower-middle classes. As industrialization increased, servitude was impractical and costly. The decline of market for home crafts, such as looming, worsened as newer industries became more productive. This obliterated the demand for the cottage work that older persons could provide. Perhaps most importantly, tenant farming or share-cropping, institutions which favor multi-generational cohabitation, were seen as increasingly inefficient. This forced many younger persons out of ancestral homesteads and eventually into the cities and factories, or to new lands.

Between approximately 1780 and 1840, in a period the social historian Charles Moranze (1957/1966) refers to as "the triumph of the middle classes," the nuclear family became the idealized norm. This was true first among the bourgeoisie, who reduced the size of their families to afford more luxuries and higher status. According to Moranze, the advent of the railroad increased wage opportunities for the lower classes who soon began to see the economic advantage of a small nuclear family.

For industrialized society the existence and popularity of the nuclear family are often seen as necessary for at least three reasons (Parsons, 1955). First, the nuclear family provides a strong work incentive. It is likely that many wage workers would have less steady employment histories if they did not have to bear responsibility for feeding children. Consequently, families as a social institution act to keep the cost of labor reduced.

Secondly, the nuclear family can provide a useful, and perhaps necessary, division of labor for additional economic productivity. This includes the tremendous amount of unpaid labor such as homemaking and community building. Until recent years this was provided almost exclusively by the wife. The absence of this unpaid source of labor is now apparent in the stress that many dual career couples face in attempting to balance homemaking and career responsibilities. Finally, the nuclear family provides a socialized source of future workers for the next generation (Parsons & Bales, 1955). The middle class has long depended upon a tradition of artisanship to achieve its economic clout. In late Medieval times, as in some professions today, occupational status was acquired after a long father-son apprenticeship. This is still common in small businesses. The nuclear family affords an extended socialization period where the roles of the parents can be satisfactorily inculcated into the next generation. This reduces the costs associated with labor role instability in an industrialized, and especially a technological society.

Today there are a number of options available to modern people other than the traditional nuclear family. More individuals are living as singles, either alone, or with groups. There is anecdotal evidence that adult siblings are living together longer and reuniting as a family following major life transitions, such as divorce. Long-term monogamous gay and lesbian relationships are common. Increasingly, society is experiencing a reuniting of parents and offspring when parents, no longer able to look after their own needs, move into their children's home. The impact that these and other changes will have on future familial and social structures is difficult to determine.

CONTEMPORARY "FAMILY PROBLEMS" AND THE RISE OF FAMILY THERAPIES

It has become almost a hackneyed expression that the (nuclear) family is "besieged," "in crisis," and "facing certain extinction." (These phrases were obtained from three consecutive articles appearing in recent popular magazines.) Concerns such as these may reflect an underlying reality, as evidenced by increasing crime, substance abuse, and changing family constellations. However, serious apprehension regarding destruction of the family as a social institution has existed since Plato. Scientific literature as early as 1927 stressed how rapid urbanization might be damaging the family as a social institution (Mowrer, 1927). Popular literature was even more explicit and placed much of the blame of "the destruction of the family" on the "menacing tide" of new immigrants to our urban areas. Many of the movies of the 1930s further inflamed the popular sentiment that the family was failing to live up to its God-appointed role (Bettmann, 1974).

The "golden age" of the family probably existed for a brief period during the late eighteenth and early nineteenth centuries. In large part, it may have been an historical fiction (Bahr, 1988). However, with a general decrease in the importance of other social institutions, such as the church and the absolute sovereignty of the state, the family has been forced to assume a more important role in socialization. This was noted by late nineteenth and early twentieth century social theorists who wondered whether an institution as new and vulnerable as the nuclear family should shoulder this burden.

Some theorists have questioned whether the contemporary institution of the family is powerful enough by itself to instill sufficient socialization experiences. It is clear that other institutions that once worked in tandem with the family are now less effective. The extended kinship and communal ties of the village family have not found a successful counterpart in the small, isolated urban household. Furthermore, beliefs that worked to regulate human behavior have lost some of their salience, such as rigid class distinctions, unquestioned theism, and strong community ties. Robert Nisbet, the prescient sociologist, noted as early as 1953 that "For many rea-

sons, the contemporary family is made to carry a conscious symbol-
ic importance that is greater than ever, but it must do this with a
structure much smaller in size and of manifestly diminishing relevance to the larger economic, religious and political ends of contemporary society" (p. 59). Nisbet, as well as many others, suggest
that the family is simply too weak for this task.

In spite of these fears, demands on the family appear to be rapidly increasing. For example, the definition of what constitutes "good
parenting" has expanded greatly in recent years (Lein, 1986). Simultaneously, parents are spending more time out of the home
working. During the last two decades families have experienced an
era of declining wages and continued inflation that forces the solo
income family into a precarious financial position. The widespread
effects of this on child socialization remain controversial and tinged
in ideology. Most family therapists, however, can recount at least
one family where the children "ran amuck" while the parents were
forced to work excessive hours.

There is also less likelihood that children will be raised in a
traditional nuclear family than in previous generations in our century. In Euro-American communities, this is due mostly to an increased divorce rate, while in African-American, and to a lesser
extent Latin American, communities it is due to both high divorce
rates and high rates of pregnancy out of wedlock. The reasons for
the latter trend remain controversial and are probably multi-deter-
mined. They include the legacy of racism, the lack of role models,
higher rates of arrest for African-American males and the stresses
of urban poverty. However, regardless of the cause, many of the
very children most in need of the advantages of a nuclear family are
denied this opportunity.

During the twentieth century, the family has undergone a quiet
and profound revolution. Wage earning classes began to marry for
"courtly" or romantic love. Regardless of the constantly encountered bond between woman and man, the present Western Euro-
pean-based notion of marriage for romantic love is a rather new
phenomenon. Romantic love has been around since recorded history
and is not, as some writers claim, an invention of our epoch. There
are numerous references to it in mythology and also biblical literature (e.g., Genesis 29: 15-30). However, as the Biblical story of

Jacob and Rachel indicates, romantic love itself was rarely an adequate reason for marriage.

As a social experiment in providing greater marital stability, marriage for romantic love is less than successful. This is clearly indicated by the increasing divorce rates. In terms of utilitarian impact, the ultimate hedonic value of romantic-based marriages is difficult to assess, since we do not know the ratio of "broken hearts" to happy lovers. Regardless, if the family is a rather flimsy base to carry the burden of socialization, romantic love is even a weaker pedestal. For many people, and despite strong expectation, romantic love simply does not last long enough. The expectations of ideal and continual marital bliss, in conjunction with the moral and economic freedom to end a conjugal relationship, place tremendous and unprecedented demands on the institution of marriage, and consequently, on the existence of the "traditional" family.

The contemporary nuclear family, then, is an institution that was born in travail and continues a difficult existence. The varieties of family therapy, including couples therapy, can be seen as attempts to mediate some of the problems between individuals and society by strengthening the socializing influences of the family.

THE HISTORY OF FAMILY THERAPY: THE DEVELOPMENTAL ANALOGY

The history of family therapy can be heuristically conceptualized through the analogy of individual psychosocial maturation. All analogies are necessarily selective; some biasing distortion is required. Yet the metaphor of personal growth may be useful for conceptualizing both the past and the future direction of family therapy theory and practice.

The Ancestors of Family Therapy

Following the rapid industrialization of the late nineteenth century the family's influence on societal stability became obvious. Scattered psychologists associated with the Functionalist school emphasized the importance of the family in preventing the burgeoning problems of a rapidly urbanizing society. Writers such as Dewey, Stark, Hall, and even William James emphasized that poverty and unstable community relations could cause delinquency or worse. Lightner Witmer's psychological clinic at the University of Pennsylvania in the late 1800s appears to have made inclusion of the family in child treatment an important goal and may have been one of the first "family-oriented" clinics. However, with the advent of both Freudianism and Behaviorism, academic psychology would do little more to pioneer family therapy for at least another fifty years.

A much greater impetus than isolated work in university-based clinics occurred in conjunction with the Child Guidance and Mental Hygiene movements of the very early twentieth century (Kaslow, 1980). These movements, which drew strength from the optimism of this period in American society, advocated that the best way to solve problems in "mental hygiene" was to prevent their occurrence. As early as 1890, social workers wrote about the need to work with the entire family of the poor together; the Child Guidance movement incorporated these ideas. "Wayward" or troubled youths at risk for social deviancy would be counseled and diverted from future instability. Better parenting would foster mentally and physically healthier children. Consequently, parental involvement in child guidance was an essential component with undetermined potential.

According to Kaslow (1980), another root of family therapy was the somewhat clandestine practice of conjugal and family intervention by practicing analysts and others. Many "avant garde" analytically oriented therapists during the 1920s and 1930s apparently practiced primitive versions of marital and family therapy. Interventions were based on an admixture of Freudian orthodoxy and common sense, probably with a good dose of moral philosophy.

Alfred Adler was one of the first theorists to systematically discuss the importance of family factors on psychopathology (Ansbacher & Ansbacher, 1956). Adler believed that most psychopathology was due to misperception of the external world, usually originating in childhood. Family factors, such as parental attitudes, birth order, or relation with siblings could cause distorted social relatedness, resulting in psychopathology.

Adlerians made several contributions to family therapy that are often overlooked. They pioneered the use of prevention of mental health problems by attempting to optimize child rearing practices. They were also among the earliest practitioners to interview families in toto, often in a public forum, since they believed that community response was therapeutic (Dreikurs, Corsini, Lowe, & Sonstegard, 1959). They also pioneered the use of extensive family history taking, including the now-popular technique of using a genogram. Adlerian family therapy continues to be popular today (Sherman & Dinkmeyer, 1987).

However, it was not until the early 1930s that the notion of autonomous theories of marital therapy became accepted. In response to the rising divorce rates that certainly would prove disastrous in the economic depression of the era, marriage counseling centers arose in major urban institutions to address these problems. Kaslow (1980) notes that these practitioners were quick to deviate from the dominant paradigm of Freudianism and attempted to experiment with new therapeutic modes suited for diadic interaction. Furthermore, instead of seeing families and spouses as potential impediments to treatment success, other family members became partners in therapy. Response from the psychodynamic community was sometimes disapproving and ostracizing. Hence, in 1942 the American Association of Marriage and Family Counselors was formed to provide an alternative forum and set of standards for practitioners working with couples and families.

The 1950s: The Birth and Childhood Years of Family Therapy

During the 1950s family therapy was "discovered" somewhat simultaneously by several individuals or groups. Excellent detailed histories are available elsewhere (Guerin, 1976; Kaslow, 1980; Olson, 1970). The present discussion will be limited to highlighting major contributions from each school to present day practice of family therapy.

Analytic Schools

One of the earliest contributors to family therapy theory and practice was Nathan Ackerman, a child psychiatrist and psychoanalyst. Ackerman was initially concerned with the fascinating area of families' behavioral changes under the stress of unemployment. Ackerman had been practicing psychiatry with unemployed miners in the 1930s and later attempted to introduce some of his ideas regarding stress and mental illness at the Menninger clinic, where he was later employed. Some accounts suggest his ideas were resoundingly criticized. However, he was able to send staff out to observe family processes in naturally occurring settings. These observations allowed him to strengthen his conclusions regarding the importance of families in the treatment of psychopathology.

Ackerman asserted that unconscious factors and past history can affect family functioning and can cause distortions in the way families relate to each other. Often these distortions are evident in the interaction between spouses. Because of the importance of historical factors, family therapy from analytic perspective involves extensive history taking, often as much as six or more sessions. Ackerman eventually opened the first family therapy training institute, in New York City. Unfortunately, he died in 1971, just as family therapy was beginning to gain its present respect.

Ackerman's principal works are available in Ackerman (1958) and in an edited volume (Ackerman, 1970). Some commentators (e.g., Goldenberg & Goldenberg, 1983) have suggested that his untimely death limited interest in psychoanalytic family therapy. However, there continues to be strong concern in the fusing of psychoanalytic/psychodynamic methods and those of family therapy, especially among analytically-oriented psychiatrists. The amalgamation of family therapy with object relations theory is also an area of current interest among this group; exemplified in the work of Framo (1982).

Simultaneously, but initially independently of Ackerman, Theodore Lidz and his associates at Yale began work in the psychoanalytic study of family processes (see Lidz, 1973, for a summary of this research). They concluded that schizophrenia was essentially a "deficiency disease" resulting, in general, from a mother with arrested personality development being unable to adequately nurture her child. Presently this concept has little empirical support, but is still popular in some circles despite its sexist attributions.

Two other contributions of this group remain important today.

Lidz and associates (Lidz, Cornelison, Fleck, & Terry, 1957; Lidz, Cornelison, Terry, & Fleck, 1958) described two types of marital discord claimed to be common in families of schizophrenics. Marital schism is open disharmony between parents, characterized by mutual undermining. Marital skew occurs when serious psychological disturbances in one parent dominate the home environment, yet the family pretends that there is no problem. (This concept is quite similar to the currently popular term "codependent household" or "codependent spouse" used frequently by substance abuse therapists). Lidz asserts that marital schism is associated with schizophrenia in daughters, while marital skew is associated with schizophrenia in sons.

John Bell, a psychologist, is often overlooked in the history of family therapy. Bell's use of families in treatment was serendipitous and has assumed an almost legendary status. While in Britain, he apparently misheard a colleague talking about John Bowlby's attachment theory-based approach to treatment of severely problematic adolescents. In 1951 Bell began interviewing the whole family together, believing this was the method that Bowlby advocated. While Bowlby did interview the entire family, he did so separately, and largely to obtain a more accurate history regarding the individual patient in treatment. Bell didn't know this and became impressed with what he thought were Bowlby's techniques because they proved successful in reducing the length of treatment. Presently, Bell espouses an approach more similar to social learning theorists than to analytic thinkers.

Transgenerational Family Therapists

Murray Bowen, an analytically trained psychiatrist, represents a bridge between analytically oriented family therapy and more novel approaches. Bowen was a pioneer of transgenerational theories of family pathology which attempt to examine the contribution of several generations of pathology to a family's present functioning. At the Menninger Clinic, and later at the National Institute of Mental Health, Bowen studied the interactive processes in families of schizophrenics. Bowen noticed a striking lack of "ego boundaries" between schizophrenics and their families. He further observed that communications were poor within these families often with one family member (usually the mother) communicating for the schizophrenic child. This research culminated in a series of studies during the mid- and late 1950s at the National Institute of Mental Health (NIMH) where entire families of schizophrenics were hospitalized together. To explain the relationship of these findings to the cause of schizophrenia and other serious mental disorders, Bowen postulated that schizophrenia is due to a lack of differentiation of self. To Bowen (1978), differentiation of self is the extent to which an individual's emotions are distinguished from their intellect. Individuals who are low on differentiation tend to view themselves and their families as a common process or "undifferentiated ego mass." Several generations of intermarriage by persons low on differentiation is hypothesized to produce a positive family history for schizophrenia, which is labelled as the "multigenerational transmission process."

Bowen has originated several other important concepts that are frequently encountered, such as "emotional cutoff," "family projection process" and "triangling." To date, he has a zealous group of followers. His influence is evident by the popularity of his concepts with practicing clinicians.

Ivan Boszormenyi-Nagy is increasingly and regrettably overlooked in accounts of the early years of family therapy. This may be because his work is often intellectually challenging to read. Boszormenyi-Nagy and his colleagues have made substantial contributions to transgenerational family therapy (e.g., Boszormenyi-Nagy & Framo, 1965). According to Boszormenyi-Nagy, family pathology is often rooted in unconscious boundaries that exist across generations. This is usually seen in the symptomatic behavior of children which is often thought to reflect unconscious parental sentiments. Because we expect life to be fair, children develop unconscious "ledgers" regarding what life owes them and what they have received. They may attempt to "balance the ledger with their own children," who may respond in turn by unconsciously acting out their parents' fantasies.

The purpose of family therapy, according to this approach, is to illuminate these ledgers and free family members of them so that symptomatic behavior can be avoided. Therapy, which is often lengthy and intensive, allows the family to secure a greater trust in each other, thereby weakening unconscious adherence to the ledgers of previous generations. A major focus of this system of therapy is the exoneration of past family members for perceived wrongdoing so that a ledger is forgiven.

Communications Theorists

Communications theorists state that the root of psychopathology is in the disturbed communication process of the family. An early theorist of this orientation was Lyman Wynne, a psychiatrist who also holds a Ph.D. in social relations from Harvard (where he studied under Talcot Parsons, the seminal sociologist). Wynne succeeded Bowen at the NIMH when Bowen went to Georgetown University. Having been trained in social relations, Wynne was especially interested in the conflicts between the needs of the child to develop an independent identity, and also the need for the development of a sense of familial intimacy (e.g. Singer & Wynne, 1965).

Wynne is responsible for two popular terms describing the family functioning of schizophrenics: pseudomutuality, and pseudohostility. The former occurs in families that appear to be functioning relatively well, yet that maintain great distance between each other. The latter occurs when families pretend to be displaying familial hostility, but actually are doing so in a much muted and ineffectual form of hostility. Schizophrenia, Wynne initially believed, was related to an individual's failure to develop a clear self-identity because of these communication distortions. As a result, the schizophrenic fails in other social situations, reinforcing involvement with the family, which further reinforces the pathology.

Wynne is a rare figure in family therapy. He combines creativity, clinical prowess and sensitivity, and a commitment to empiricism. Unlike many other family therapists, he has not shied away from criticizing his own notions if they have not been supported by data. He continues to refine his concepts of family risk factors for schizophrenia. Wynne was also among the first among his peers to recognize the growing and hostile gap between family therapists and parents of those with major mental illness who resented being blamed (and by some therapists, being seen as the sole cause) for their childrens' conditions. By advocating that family therapists assume a consultational and allied role with parents, he may have averted the major confrontation between family therapy practitioners and victims advocates that seemed inevitable during the early 1980s.

The best known communication theorists were the group associated with Gregory Bateson at Palo Alto Veterans Affairs (then Veterans Administration) Hospital during the 1950s. Bateson was initially attracted to Norbert Weiner's theory of cybernetics, popular immediately following World War II. In conjunction with a creative group (Jay Haley, a graduate student in communications, John Weakland, a former chemical engineer, and Don Jackson, a psychiatrist) Bateson began to explore the relation between paradoxical language and schizophrenia.

In 1956 the group published the "double bind" theory of schizophrenia (Bateson, Jackson, Haley, & Weakland, 1956). Essentially, double bind messages are those that are internally contradictory, such as when a parent slaps a child and states "I love you." Contradiction can exist solely on a verbal level, such as when someone states, "I always lie." More often, contradictions occur between verbal and nonverbal content, as illustrated in the example above or when a parent disconfirms a verbal message with strong and contradictory nonverbal communications. A parent who grimaces while telling a child how much she is loved is an example of the latter case. For a communication to be considered double bind it must also be received from an emotionally important person to the listener and be structured so that it cannot be disallowed. Bateson's group proposed that exposure to repeated double bind messages is an important ingredient in the causation of schizophrenia.

By the late 1950s the Palo Alto group began to separate. Jackson formed the Mental Research Institute (MRI) in Palo Alto, where Haley was associated for a time. Then in 1962, Ackerman, Jackson, and Haley founded the first family therapy journal, *Family Process*. Haley became interested in the works of the psychiatrist/hypnotherapist Milton Erikson, and subsequently edited Erikson's collected papers. Eventually, Haley left California for a productive association with Salvador Minuchin in Philadelphia, and later founded his own training institute in Washington, D.C. Jackson died in 1967 and Weakland remained with MRI. He continues his pioneering work in brief, problem focused therapies. Much of this work has strongly influenced the treatment strategies with resistant families that he advocates in this volume.

Humanistic Theorists

Virginia Satir, a social worker by training, was referred to Don Jackson by Murray Bowen, whom she had sought out because of her similar work with families. Satir became associated with the MRI, where she advocated a very popular form of family therapy (Satir, 1967; 1972) that was a mixture of Gestalt psychology, communication theory, and popular techniques of the 1960s such as encounter therapies. She also advanced the Growth Potential Movement, Sensitivity Awareness, Encounter Groups, and Gestalt Psychology at Esalen Institute with Fritz Perls.

Carl Whitaker, a charismatic psychiatrist, began working extensively with couples in the late 1950s. Whitaker coined the phrase "experiential psychotherapy" while working on the East Coast in the 1950s. Much of his Zen-like technique is impossible to separate from his irreverent personal style. Although lacking a theoretically consistent set of beliefs regarding family therapy, he is best categorized as a Humanist. He advocated "craziness" and nonrational thought on the part of both the family and the therapist.

Cybernetics

Despite genuine differences, many of the family therapists during this period were united in their emphasis that cybernetic processes operate to maintain family stability. The word cybernetics is derived from the Greek word meaning, "the science of steering ships." The term was popularized as the result of a book by Norbert Weiner in 1948, based in part on a previous work by Weiner, Artureo Rosenblueth, and Julian Bigelow. Both Weiner and an early proponent of cybernetics, W. R. Ashby, viewed cybernetics primarily as a science of machines, with the application of these principles into areas of biophysics, molecular biology, and other fields of secondary importance. In more recent years, the term cybernetics has narrowed to describe how the analogy of certain systems common to machines can be applied to living organisms. Family therapists who state that families "function cybernetically" often mistakenly believe that they are claiming that families function similar to living organisms.

Cybernetics involves the way machines use information to maintain a desired output. Many of the notions of cybernetics can be traced to the ancients. In more modern times, authors such as Descartes, La Mettrie, and T. H. Huxley argued that life forms behave similarly to machines. Clerk Maxwell, the physicist, presented the first scientific account of the role of feedback mechanisms in physical behavior in an 1868 paper entitled "On governance." Many nineteenth century sociologists also incorporated rudimentary notions of feedback into their conceptions of society.

However, the true beginnings of cybernetics can be credited to the years of World War II. By this time, a number of machines, both electrical and mechanical, had been developed to restrict or increase output to a desired level, based on previous feedback. For our discussion, there are two important types of feedback loops or processes. Positive feedback loops amplify output to a desired level, such as when the smaller current passing through a vacuum tube or transistor modifies a larger but unmodulated current to produce a much greater output. Negative feedback loops act to dampen deviations from a set point, such as when a thermostat turns on the heat to raise the temperature. Wiener, Ashby, and others put forth what has come to be known as "the cybernetic hypothesis," namely that the properties of living systems can be fruitfully studied by applying the principles of information flow in machines.

A notion central to cybernetics is the concept of homeostasis, or maintenance of a steady state (von Bertalanffy, 1968). First popularized by the physiologist Walter Cannon, homeostasis refers to the process by which organisms maintain a consistent internal environment despite varying external conditions. Without homeostasis organisms would quickly die. Even standing up from a chair would cause a precipitous drop in blood pressure which might prove fatal. Usually, homeostatic mechanisms function by a series of negative feedback loops (Gray & Rizzo, 1969).

Sociologists of the functional school argue that social institutions, including the family, strive to maintain a steady state. Many family therapists have adapted these ideas to clinical theory by arguing that homeostatic mechanisms, particularly negative feedback mechanisms, maintain dysfunctional or symptomatic behaviors in families. For example, in the classic formulation of the substance abuse "enabler," the abusive drinking by one spouse triggers compensatory behaviors by the other spouse designed to smooth over any problems that may affect the family unit. This acts to decrease the consequences of substance abuse to both the user and family.

The first extensive clinical discussion of cybernetic processes involving family regulation was advanced by Jackson (1957). Jackson proposed that a series of homeostatic mechanisms within the family serves to regulate the behavior of the family's members. Clinical experience suggested to him that one or more family members often functioned as a thermostat, deviating from routine behavior when excessive destabilizing forces were acting within or upon the family system. The results of this thermostatic action were to return the family system to its previous level of stability. Dysfunctional behavior on the part of a family member was therefore seen as a "safety valve," actually encouraging family system stability.

The belief that homeostatic mechanisms maintain family processes imbued family therapists with incredible optimism regarding the process of behavioral change. From this discussion of homeostasis, we can see that it seems likely that an increase in functional behavior of the family system will be reinforced and maintained by homeostatic mechanisms in the family, just as much as the dysfunctional behavior was once maintained. Simply change the behavior, and the family will ensure that the change is maintained.

Cybernetic family feedback may also yield negative consequences for the family. As Kantor and Lehr (1975) note, excessive feedback can result in a system being closed to outside experience, and hence unable to satisfactorily and proactively adjust to changes in the environment. In cybernetic theory, the closed system cannot incorporate additional information beyond its limited system of negative feedbacks. Satir (1967) was the first to popularize the notion that negative feedback loops can be stifling for family growth, or even for the capacity of families to cope with life. Satir saw the behavior of some families as synonymous with closed cybernetics systems. These families were incapable of incorporating positive feedback from new experiences, and consequently were restricted and threatened by their environment. We can predict that such families are very likely to terminate therapy, primarily because they are threatened by the prospects of change.

Family Therapy During the 1960s and 1970s: An Adolescence

As Goldenberg and Goldenberg (1983) note, the field of family therapy in the 1960s was characterized by a "rush to practice." No one technique predominated, although the dominant implicit theoretical stance adopted by most therapists was that dysfunctional behavior was to be viewed as the product of dysfunctional relationships, rather than individual pathology. The term "identified patient" (IP) (Haley, 1976) became immensely popular as family therapists postulated that the IP was merely a "symptom bearer" for the family's composite problems. This sentiment was best expressed by Satir (1967) who stated that a person's individual symptoms were the message that he or she is being forced to distort personal growth in order to divert family pain.

During this period there was much optimism regarding the therapeutic efficacy of family therapy that was based on very little data or even theory. Perhaps this is related to the enthusiasm that American society displayed in attempting to eliminate its social problems during this period. Family therapy seemed a natural method to correct problems of poverty, the cycle of illiteracy and underachievement, and even racism. Family therapy was frequently used as adjunctive to the popular community psychiatry movement of this period, where indigenous community leaders and paraprofessionals were often touted as superior to trained practitioners in providing services for poor and minority community residents. The attempts at serious scientific scholarship by family therapists during this period were rare with the exception of the work of Salvador Minuchin and his group (e.g., Minuchin & Montalvo, 1967; Minuchin, Montalvo, Guerney, Rosman, & Schudmer, 1967; Minuchin, Rosman & Baker, 1978). In response to concern regarding chronic family dysfunctionality among ghetto residents, Minuchin and associates scrutinized the structure of poor urban families. Of 12 families of delinquent children studied, more than three-quarters had no stable father figure. These families were characterized by sparse communication and little sibling interaction. Two types of family structures were found to be common: the enmeshed family, with individual overinvolvement in other family members' lives, and the disengaged family in which parents virtually abdicated appropriate authority.

Minuchin's work represents some of the first outcome literature in family therapy. Furthermore, his work with "high risk" families allowed him time to refine both theory and technique. In 1965 he became director of the Philadelphia Child Guidance Clinic where he collaborated with Haley. There, Minuchin and Haley pioneered what is now known as structural family therapy, since a primary goal of therapy is creation and maintenance of an adequate family hierarchy or structure. An excellent description of this theory and its related techniques is available in Minuchin (1974).

However, like other adolescents, family therapy during this period engaged in braggadocio, if not self-deception. During this stage many practitioners espoused an anti-empirical, and even an anti-theoretical, stance. Other practitioners asserted, with little or no scientific evidence, that family therapy was the sole treatment of choice for every psychiatric disorder. The results in some cases were disastrous, as when some family practitioners told schizophrenics and patients with severe affective disorders to discontinue psychopharmacological treatment. In other clinics individuals without cooperative or geographically available families were excluded from treatment completely. In still others, severe though treatable problems, such as manic depressive illness, were glossed over as "merely symptoms" of "deeper" family problems.

The Late 1970s and 1980s: Young Adulthood

There are surprisingly few theoretical models in the behavioral science literature addressing the process by which individuals pass from the storm of adolescence to maturity. Young adulthood is a necessary intermediary step, where the excesses of adolescence, tempered by valuable experience, are reconsidered and delimited. It is a time of consolidation and self-reflection, where abilities are subjectively weighed and longer-term goals are established. Invariably, it involves extensive self-inquiry and subsequent behavioral change. Parallels can be found regarding the development of family therapy.

According to Goldenberg and Goldenberg (1983), the history of family therapy in the 1970s and 1980s involved two trends: increasing self-examination and increased professionalization. Self-examination included a long-needed scrutiny of the efficacy of therapeutic techniques. Writers such as Olson, Russell, and Sprenkle (1980) argued that for family therapy to mature as a field it must be able to authenticate its efficacy through consistent high quality research. The empirical literature that did exist up to that time was generally poorly designed, and often did not include pre- and post-treatment measures of change. By the mid-1980s a number of research articles, including meta-analyses, indicated the efficacy of family therapy. Despite occasional claims from responsible theoreticians that research is irrelevant, impractical, or even logically impossible, the prevailing sentiment today is that family therapy should be rooted at least ideally in both art and science, and therefore should be based upon replicable results (L'Abate, 1986).

Self-examination also involved increasing self-criticism regarding precise definition of terms and theoretical development. Practitioners from the mid-1970s onward have been more careful to describe their techniques, illustrating the use of their methods through extensive case reporting. An advantage of more comprehensive descriptions of family therapy now available in the literature is that they are more apt to hold greater explanatory power to nonfamily therapists who are in a position to recommend families for treatment (McCown & Johnson, 1985). Furthermore, descriptions facilitate replication of purported results and hasten the learning process of therapists-in-training.

The Maturation of Family Therapy

Presently, there are a number of competing "schools" or general approaches to family intervention.

It is clear to even the casual observer that there is substantial disagreement between practitioners regarding appropriate theory and methods of family therapy. Some view this as unfortunate, while others regard it as a source of innovation and creativity (L'Abate, 1986). Regardless, the next generation promises a greater fusion between advocates of different theoretical persuasions. This is evident in a number of publications that attempt to combine theoretical approaches.

Issues concerning the quality of family therapy research have been raised since the 1980s. Psychotherapy research is complex; family therapy research even more so (Todd & Stanton, 1983). Unfortunately, it appears that many family therapists are still woefully unprepared to formulate and execute the rather technical research that is increasingly necessary. Ideally, if practitioners are not trained to be researchers they should at least be taught to be intelligent consumers of research literature. This additional training will probably involve a greater sophistication in research methods than many present day practitioners possess.

As indicated by the large number of specialty publications, there appears to be a growing sentiment that a single theoretical technique for family intervention, or even single theory, is inadequate. As we will argue in later chapters, family therapy with resistant systems may require different techniques and theories. This observation is an extension of the question proposed by Paul (1967) regarding individual therapy outcome: what type of therapy works best for what kind of family under what conditions. We hope this question will soon be answered by data rather than conjecture. However, the development of theory and technique must logically precede the testing of theory and technique.

Numerous books have been written to describe theories and techniques of different contemporary schools of family therapy. Excellent general introductions are provided by several authors, and virtually all of the "classic" texts in family therapy are still easily available and are surprisingly readable. These include Ackerman (1970), Boszormenyi-Nagy and Framo (1965) (more challenging reading), Bowen (1978), Framo (1982), Haley (1976; 1980), Minuchin (1974), and Satir (1967). Numerous and more specialized texts yield surveys of particular schools and are also very useful.

THE FUTURE OF FAMILY THERAPY:
DYNAMICAL SYSTEMS THEORY

Since the inception of family therapy, therapists have been concerned with nonlinear processes of stability and change (Guerin,
1976). Although the impact of general systems theory on other
sciences has only been moderate (von Bertalanffy, 1968), its impact
on family theorists and practitioners has been substantial. It has
become almost a cliché for the family therapist to state that he or
she thinks "systemically" about a family's behavior. However, it is
likely many more therapists purport to "think systemically" than
actually understand systems theory. For example, "systemic thinking" is occasionally used as a rationale for vague speculation about
a family's functioning or as an apology for careless or indecisive
family interventions. At other times the art of family therapy has
gone beyond the language of science to describe the impact of
interventions upon systemic functioning.

During the last 20 years there has been a revolution in the understanding of nonlinear systems (Gleick, 1987). This paradigm shift
has been loosely described as "chaos theory," or perhaps more
appropriately, dynamical systems theory (Abraham, Abraham, &
Shaw, 1991). These developments provide a better language for
descriptions of complex systems, and an improved understanding of
nonlinear processes of complex systems such as family functioning.
Developments within chaos theory also offer a simplified way of
viewing extraordinarily complex systems, ranging from the behavior of molecules to the functioning of economic forces in society.

The concepts within dynamical systems theory are similar to the
assumptions of many family therapists (Chamberlain, 1991). Abraham, Abraham, and Shaw (1991) summarize many of the key concepts of chaos theory. The first assumption is that instead of being
viewed as events to be explained, systems are viewed as complex
evolving relationships. Systems are dynamic, rather than static. Consequently, a study of systems necessitates the study of change as well
as stability. This notion is almost identical to a number of systems
theorist thinkers, including Jackson's (1957) account of the necessity
of studying family homeostatic processes, Satir's (1967) emphasis
on family dynamics, and Haley's (1976) emphasis on family change.

The second assumption found in dynamical systems theory is that the behavior of all systems can be modeled through an essential set of rules, usually differential equations. Although few family therapists have explored the mathematics involved in the behavior of family systems, many have emphasized the unwritten or verbalized rules in the family and their effects on systemic functioning. These include practically all of the structural/strategic theorists, as well as theorists such as Ackerman (1970), Boszormenyi-Nagy and Framo (1965), Bowen (1978) and Zuck (1971).

The third assumption is that causality is considered multileveled and multidetermined. Parts of the system influence each other, which in turn influence other systemic aspects. This has been one of the tenets of family therapy since its beginning (Guerin, 1976) and is probably what separates family therapists from their less systemically oriented colleagues.

A fourth feature of dynamical systems theory involves the concept of "self-organization." This constitutes one of the contributions of chaos theory that does not have a clear parallel in current family therapy theory. Self-organization refers to the idea that the behavior of a system is influenced by feedback from its previous behavior. Such a system is said to possess "self-control." A classic example drawn from population biology occurs when the previous year's population levels influence the following year's population values. This example illustrates the potential complexities in nondynamical systems modeling. If population values of a given animal group (such as rabbits) are low during the first year, the second year may see an increase in the population, as there is less competition for food. However, if population values are too low, the population may face excessive pressure from predators such as foxes, and therefore extinction. Similarly, a high population of rabbits may be associated with lesser numbers the next year, due to starvation and disease, unless the elevated population causes sating of the predators, in which case the population may rise further. All of these complexities can be modeled mathematically with differential (i.e., nonlinear) equations.

As a corollary of self-organization, feedback is extraordinarily important for future behavior. Even small variations in initial conditions and feedback values can have enormous influence on systemic functioning. Another implication of self-organization is that perfect homeostasis of systems is neither necessarily optimal nor ever completely possible, an assumption suggested earlier by Satir (1967) and other humanistic family therapists. Homeostasis is often variable, rather than an absolute level.

A related and critical feature of dynamical systems theory is that chaos, or seemingly random behavior that differs substantially from previous functioning, is a ubiquitous and perfectly natural phenomenon of complex systems (Marks, 1991). The behavior of systems can be stable or undergo gradual changes most of the time, only to be punctuated by dramatic changes in systemic functioning called bifurcations. Extreme fluctuations following bifurcation are called chaotic states. Often, a more advantageous systemic functioning follows periods of chaos.

It is important to realize that systems fluctuating from a state of stability to chaos can be stabilized in two ways. One obvious way is to provide more homeostatic restrictive feedback. For example, we can control the population of rapidly breeding rabbits by introducing more hunters or natural predators, thereby ensuring that population values for future years fall within a more narrow range. A less intuitive way of stabilizing wildly fluctuating systems is to *add noise*. Although we cannot discuss the mathematics of adding noise to oscillating systems here, our rabbit and fox analogy may be helpful if not taken too literally. The population of rabbits can be stabilized if other parameters of the system are varied randomly, such as disease rates, food supply, available territory, and predators.

Chaos theory has already been applied to descriptions of family functioning (Elkaim, Goldber, & Goldbeter-Merinfeld, 1987). Indeed, Chamberlain (1991) believes the language of chaos theory will provide better models of family stability and instability, eventually unifying many of the presently popular competing approaches to family systems theory. This becomes clear when comparing the structural approaches of Minuchin and his associates with the humanistic interventions of Satir and Whitaker. Structural approaches can be primarily viewed as serving to increase restrictive or negative homeostatic feedback with subsequent reduction in an oscillating system's potential for chaos. In contrast, humanistic therapies may provide more noise to the system, stabilizing it by employing entirely different techniques. Strategic therapy approaches attempt a delicate balancing act of providing feedback and simultaneously increasing noise.

It is our belief that the various schools of family therapy may soon be united by an increasing emphasis on nonlinear dynamical systems theory. Whether chaos theory will be a more accurate model of family functioning or simply a useful heuristic remains to be determined. Regardless, many of the concepts of this rapidly expanding paradigm of science seem to have direct applicability to clinical work with families. The present volume will illustrate several of these applications and their relevance to the therapy of resistant family systems. However, our understanding of chaos theory is quite limited and our interventions may be more analogous than truly theory-driven. It is almost certain that the next generation of researchers and clinicians will improve upon our ignorance of the family as a dynamical system.

Chapter Three

Family Resistance, Stress, and Crises

RESISTANCE AND CRISIS INTERVENTION

Our central contention is that therapy with treatment resistant families often necessitates the techniques of crisis intervention. There are several reasons for this. Treatment resistance is inextricably linked with family crises. Resistant families are often introduced to therapy only after there is a significant disruption in their system. These families are likely to terminate treatment within just a few sessions, even before their initial crisis is resolved. A task of therapy with these families is to keep them in treatment long enough to experience some benefit. Simultaneously, it is important that the therapist proceed with caution and not harm the family by interventions that may inappropriately destabilize the system should the family terminate abruptly and prematurely. Hence, the therapist needs to proceed cautiously and with these considerations in mind.

Resistant families are also often crisis-prone. We label these families as "high risk systems" because they are at very high risk to terminate therapy abruptly and then to subsequently present during another crisis. When families are both treatment resistant and crisis-prone they represent particular difficulties for both themselves and treatment providers. The task with these families is to effectively manage the present crisis but in such a way as to avoid premature termination of treatment once the immediate crisis is resolved.

The family system's response to internal and external stressors mediates the relation between resistance and crisis. Various responses include the family's perception of stress, reaction to this perception, and the system's coping mechanisms. These three classes of variables combine to determine whether a family will be treatment resistant, high risk, crisis-prone but cooperative, or within normal limits regarding propensity for both treatment resistance and crisis-proneness.

This chapter will review some of the theories regarding family crisis, stress, and coping. We will then introduce a new typology of stress, based upon the objective potential seriousness of the stressor to permanently disrupt the family. Important implications of these variables for the manner in which the family responds to initial sessions of family therapy will be presented. Finally, we will consider variables influencing family homeostasis following a crisis and use this information to formulate an intervention strategy for dealing with highly resistant and crisis-prone systems.

CRISES AND STRESSORS

Crisis theory deals with the disruption and response óf the individual or a system following a crisis situation (Moos & Schaeffer, 1986). The implicit paradigm found in most crisis theory is that crises interrupt personal, familial, or societal homeostatic mechanisms. A basic tenet is that crises are self-limiting (Caplan, 1964) inasmuch as individuals or systems cannot remain in a state of disequilibrium or emotional disarray for an indefinite amount of time. Hence, resolution to the crisis must occur at some point. Along these lines, crises are said to present opportunity, because a new and more optimal adjustment may emerge out of this disequilibrium.

The potential for crises to promote either a growth experience or have permanent adverse effects on functioning has long been noted in the family sociology literature. For example, the roller coaster model of family adjustment is a clever metaphor for both the positive and negative possibilities of change following familial exposure to severe stress. According to the model, a sufficiently severe stressor may precipitate family crisis, defined as a period of disorganization. During this time frame, previous coping strategies are inoperable, blocked, or inadequate. Eventually, the family reverses this disorganization and begins a process of recovery. Finally, the family may reach a new level of reorganization or adaptation because of the crisis.

Chaos Theory, discussed in Chapter Two, provides a supplemental framework for understanding family crises. Chaos theory suggests that homeostasis is only one of many potential states of a system (Marks, 1991). Periods of chaos, rather than homeostasis, are common in most, if not all systems. Systems with relatively weak negative feedback mechanisms may be more likely than others to experience frequent chaotic periods. If chaos is assumed to be analogous to family functioning during extreme crises, the superior reorganization of families following crisis periods is more readily explained. Chaotic systems frequently resolve into a period of superior self-control and stability without external intervention.

If the family is fortunate, its reorganization will allow a higher level of functioning than maintained prior to the experience of the stress. In other words, the crisis will have allowed for familial growth. Often, however, families never recover from severe stressors. In this case, the family's functioning will be impaired relative to functioning prior to the experience of the stressor. Chaos, or periodicity, rather than homeostasis will characterize the systems behavior.

Many clinicians' knowledge of the dynamics of family crises seems to end with the roller coaster model. For the family therapist this is particularly unfortunate since much of family therapy involves crisis intervention, regardless of the family's history. In order to facilitate an understanding of the impact stress and crises have on subsequent family behavior, we need to first discuss current research regarding stress and stressors.

Anyone who has experienced a personal crisis can quickly attest that crisis situations involve stress. But what is stress, and how is it related to crises? Before we can answer the latter question we must address the first, and this has proven much more complex than it might seem.

A universally satisfactory definition of stress and stressors has eluded researchers in the field. This is true despite the fact that the past fifty years has yielded an elaborate and complex literature on the topic. Theorists have focused on stress at a cellular, biological-systemic, individual, family, community and even a national level. Not surprisingly, given the breadth of focus, there has been little consensus regarding the meaning of the term.

Although the model of physiological adaptation suggested by Seyle (1956) has been found to be somewhat inaccurate, this popular theory of the causes and effects of stress remains prevalent among stress theorists and many clinicians. One reason for this is because the theory holds considerable heuristic value. Seyle, a physiologist, defined stress as an organism's experience of a physiologically arousing event, or a change. Since individuals have idiosyncratic needs for stimulation, current life stressors can vary depending upon the individual, and thus range from insufficient to optimal to excessive. Despite this, excessive stress is typically noxious, and usually precipitates an adaptive reaction in the body. Briefly, this reaction involves the secretion of many neurohormones that have the ultimate effect of expediting the process of adaptation.

Seyle argues that organisms demonstrate a continuum of adaptation in response to stress. Seyle introduced the now well-known belief that exhaustion and collapse are the inevitable outcome of prolonged adaptation to excessive stressors. Eventually, the organism's adaptive capacities are expended and the organism is overcome by the stressors. Usually, this means death, or at least dysfunctionality of the stressed system.

According to many stress theorists, stress becomes a crisis when the organism's usual response repertoire is ineffective at maintaining control over the environment. Crises can be provoked by a number of subjective stressors that accumulate until effective responding is prevented. In this case, first noted by Seyle, the organism becomes too exhausted to respond adequately. Each additional stressor can jeopardize the probability the organism will respond appropriately to control the stress. Or, the organism can subjectively perceive that active responses would be ineffectual in controlling the stressor.

From this viewpoint, we argue that crises represent a position on the continuum of response to excessive stress. Crises are not dichotomous, but instead represent a process that is subject to considerable variations. Individuals or families who are faced with extreme stressors may vary in their capacity to cope, even on a moment-by-moment basis. Consequently, their degree of incapacitation from a stressor may fluctuate considerably over even short intervals of time. Clinically, they may appear to be waxing in and out of a crisis, depending upon their momentary ability to access the necessary resources to cope. We refer to individuals and families in this predicament as being "in a crisis modality."

However, as stressors increase, the likelihood that individuals or families will be less able to cope also increases. Ultimately, we believe, every individual and family has a level of stress that will precipitate a crisis. It is important to identify factors related to this critical level of familial stress. As we will argue later in the chapter, we believe these factors relate to the extent to which a family system is crisis-prone.

FAMILY STRESS

People and families are both cybernetic systems. This suggests that both families and individuals are subjected to similar stress processes. Thus, the distinction between individual and familial response to stress is somewhat artificial. Whatever happens to the individual also happens to the family, unless homeostatic mechanisms within the family system act to mediate the effects.

However, in addition to being an aggregate of people, most theorists agree that families possess systemic properties that can magnify and/or decrease the results of stress on individual members. A much higher level of total stress is usually thought necessary to disrupt the functional family than is necessary to disrupt the individual (Parsons, 1955). An example of this concept is illustrated in the instance where families continue to function even upon the death of a member.

Despite the decreased vulnerability commonly seen in higher systems, the family itself may be subjected to particular stresses beyond those of its individual members. A definition of family stress needs to incorporate the reciprocal interaction between personal and familial events (Landau-Stanton & Stanton, 1985). Not surprisingly, such a definition of family stress has proven difficult and occasionally controversial. Therefore, it is best to be conservative. Our definition is by no means the only one available, nor is it necessarily all-inclusive. However, it is one that many family therapists would endorse. Family stress is defined as an "upset in the steady state of the family," a definition suggested by Boss (1988), a principal family stress theorist. This is also a definition congruent with the systems orientation of most family therapists.

We can also define family stress by its consequences to the family system. In this framework, a family stress is defined as a life event or occurrence that is of sufficient magnitude to precipitate a change in the family system (Hill, 1949). Note that this stress can primarily and initially affect one, several, or all of the entire family members, either individually or simultaneously. Taken together, these definitions clarify the relation of individual stress to that of the family. When stress on an individual family member produces an upset in the steady state of the family, then the stress is also familial in nature.

Note the similarities between these definitions and Seyle's definition of stress as an organismic change. In response to stressors–i.e., change–families will display the continuum of adaptation suggested by Seyle. If the stressors extend beyond the family's coping ability, the family will then become dysfunctional and may eventually collapse. In the language of dynamical systems theory, these families will behave chaotically.

TYPOLOGIES OF FAMILY STRESSORS

Boss (1988) provides a useful typology of family stressors. This typology is based on three constructs: Type, Source, and Severity. The definition of severity is self-evident inasmuch as some crises are clearly more severe than others. In our experience, however, this dimension is sometimes overlooked by clinicians who may tend to treat all stresses as equal in their capacity to precipitate family disruption.

Boss conceptualizes the distinction of stressor *type* as composed of five nonorthogonal (i.e., related) dimensions. Maturational stresses are those that come about predictably due to natural processes. In contrast, situational stressors are due to a specific episode or life event. Adolescence or senescence are examples of a maturational family stress while criminal victimization constitutes a situational stress.

Normative stresses are defined by Boss as stress associated with the normal losses and gains to family membership. This contrasts with the sudden loss of a member from an accident or natural disaster. The birth of a child is a normative stress, as is the death of an elderly parent. Sudden losses occur less frequently, but include any sudden death of a family member.

Developmental stressors are those that originate within the organism, whereas environmental stressors are peripheral and imposed from external factors. The routine tensions between parents and growing children that erupt into occasional family skirmishes are an example of developmental stresses. Environmental stresses include those in the community, such as crime, lack of economic opportunity, or the possibility of exposure to environmental toxins. Some authors have noted that a combination of developmental stressors can make families less resilient to environmental stressors (Estrella, 1988; Pittman, 1973; Todd, 1988).

Predictable stressors, as the name implies, are able to be anticipated. Often, they are related to developmental family cycles (Carter & McGoldrick, 1980). Unpredictable stressors are much more difficult to manage, partially because they leave no time to develop adequate coping strategies. We will discuss the role of stress predictability at length later.

Finally, volitional stressors involve stress encountered in pursuit of another goal. These stresses are voluntarily assumed, at least in part. Nonvolitional stressors are events that the family cannot control. When a spouse quits work to attend graduate school, the family stressors are said to be volitional. When a spouse quits work because of the manifestations of advanced HIV disease, the stressors that the family suffer are nonvolitional.

RESPONSES TO NORMATIVE
AND CATASTROPHIC STRESSORS

Following Hill's seminal formulation (1949), Boss further classifies the source of stress. Stress that emanates from *within* the family is usually less threatening than stress from outside the family. Stressors from within the family include a variety of potential events, such as having a child with a drug problem. Examples of stressful family events from outside the family are primarily environmental stressors, such as the effects of war, hurricanes, or crime.

A slightly different classification is favored by other family stress theorists. McCubbin and Figley's (1983) work highlights the distinction between normative and catastrophic stresses. Normative or transitional stresses are changes that occur in the family due to maturation and internal processes. An example is the effects of the adolescent on the family. Catastrophic stresses are sudden and extreme, and are usually viewed as a threat to survival. This distinction between normative and catastrophic stressors has been given additional impetus by the attention that family therapists are now conferring to the potential of normative family stresses in challenge to family function (Falicov, 1988).

McCubbin and Figley argue that the two types of stress differ quantitatively and qualitatively on at least 11 dimensions. Table 3.1 illustrates these differences:

TABLE 3.1. Normative and Catastrophic Stress: How They Differ

1. *Time to Prepare.* Normative stresses generally afford some time for preparation. Catastrophic stresses offer little or no such preparation time.
2. *Degree of Anticipation.* Normative family stresses generally can be anticipated. An example is the birth of a baby. Catastrophic stress is less predictable, such as the advent of a hurricane.
3. *Previous Experience.* Families often have previous experience with normative stressors. For example, the stress from a particularly unruly adolescent may be heralded by a lesser but similar experience with one of the adolescent's siblings. Catastrophic experiences usually afford no warning.
4. *Sources of Guidance.* Families have a wealth of resources to advise them about "family problems" such as teen pregnancy, childhood toilet training, or transition to first schooling experience. Families have few, if any, sources of guidance for dealing with catastrophic stresses.
5. *Experience by Others.* Families have many models for dealing with normative stressors, but few regarding catastrophic stressors.
6. *Time.* Normative family stressors purportedly do not last as long as catastrophic stressors.

7. *Sense of Control and Helplessness.* Figley and McCubbin argue that families feel less out of control during normalized stressors, compared with catastrophic events.
8. *Sense of Disruption and Destruction.* Generally, normative stressors risk fewer permanent disruptions to the family than catastrophic stressors.
9. *Degree of Danger.* Catastrophic stressors imply a higher degree of physical danger.
10. *Degree of Associated Emotional Problems.* Normative family stressors rarely cause permanent emotional problems. Extreme or catastrophic stressors may precipitate numerous and permanent increases in symptomatology.
11. *Degree of Compounding Medical Problems.* Normative family stressors rarely cause severe psychosomatic medical conditions, such as hypertension, headaches, tachycardia, insomnia, or asthma. These and other conditions are sometimes found following catastrophic stress.

After McCubbin and Figley, 1983.

PERCEPTUAL AND INSTRUMENTAL STRESSES: AN ALTERNATIVE FORMULATION

Although we find the previous categorizations and observations highly useful for clinical practice, they fail to conceptualize the enormous differences families have in response to various stresses. The novice family therapist quickly learns that families possess tremendous variation in what is considered by them to be a crisis. Some families react to normative stressors as if they were extremely traumatic. Other families, apparently more resilient ones, react to traumatic or catastrophic stressors as if they were completely controllable and simply minor developmental phases.

Crises differ both qualitatively and quantitatively in their degree of objective seriousness. Just as stressors can be aligned onto a continuum of normative versus traumatic, stresses can be described by an underlying dimension of objective seriousness. The following two cases, telephone calls to an emergency worker in a Community Mental Health Center, illustrate the differences:

Family Study 3.1. The Lawtons

> Mr. Ernest Lawton, a 41-year-old business executive and father of three called stating that he needed an emergency appointment.
>
> "It's that trashy son of mine. How the hell could he be a son of mine? All the other kids, all my kids, are fine, you know? I've got three of them and they're all fine. All doing fine. But that goddamn Eric . . . You wouldn't believe it. His insolence! (Angrily) I told him last year, 'Look, you're 14. It's time you start thinking about getting your grades up. No more, C's, okay?' And what does he do? (Extremely angrily) On his next, very next report card he gets two A's, two B's and two C's! I could kill that little punk. Two C's! Doesn't he listen to his father? Godalmighty, can you believe it? It's like he didn't hear a damn word I said to him! I laid down the law and he didn't hear me . . . You've got to talk some sense into him . . . It's been two weeks since he got that damn report card, and I'm madder now than I ever was."

While we can be relatively certain that the family's problems are broader than Eric's last report card, it is difficult for the therapist to believe that there is much immediate need to this caller's pleas. Certainly, the caller is quite upset. He seems to have reached a "breaking point." But the therapist who answers this call may be forced to wonder, quite frankly, what's the emergency? Why did he call *now*? Contrast the seeming degree of seriousness of this call with the next one, received only several minutes later by the same crisis worker:

Family Study 3.2. The Dawes

> Catherine Dawes, a 39-year-old homemaker, called in a very "flat," almost disoriented state. She spoke matter-of-factly, with little emotion. "I need some information. Some help . . . maybe you can give me some advice . . . My husband just died of a heart attack. It was, well, it was completely unexpected. I'm at the hospital. I don't know what to do next.

It was–it was quick–and I . . . I think he made his peace with God before he went. So, I can accept it, you know. I mean, I feel when it's your time, it's okay.

"But how do I tell the children? My 17-year-old daughter just got out of the hospital for depression. She tried to kill herself and her dad and I put her in _____. I need to tell her soon. But I know she'll blame herself. I'm afraid of what she'll do then. I don't have the slightest idea what to do. Can you help me?"

These two examples represent extremes. They indicate that some stressors and the subsequent crises they evoke seem more apparent and easier to empathize with than others. This empathy is based upon the degree of objective severity the crisis appears to possess. It is easy to empathize with the devastation Mrs. Dawes must feel with the death of her husband. It is much harder to empathize with the anger Mr. Lawton feels towards Eric. This is especially true since Mr. Lawton's anger towards his son's report card had reached its pinnacle many days following the report card's first appearance.

Yet Mr. Lawton is clearly upset, even livid. Later in the evening, he would smash several items of furniture in his living room and physically threaten his son. On the other hand, Mrs. Dawes would cope exceptionally well with the obviously devastating crisis she faced. She and her children would begin the arduous task of rebuilding their shattered lives. The irony in the above examples is that the most severe adjustment problems were associated with the least serious crisis.

A disparity between the perception of the stress by the participants and the actual seriousness of the stress occurs commonly in clinical practice. Sometimes, this involves cases where the participants in a severe stress or crisis deny the severity of their circumstances. This commonly follows a catastrophic stressor. Usually, however, the clinician encounters individuals and families that seem to overreact to minor stress-evoking events. Many of the "crises" that family therapists routinely handle really seem to be pseudo-crises and some family therapists refer to them as such. They are situations where it is initially difficult to understand exactly why the family system is facing a challenge. Or, perhaps, they are situations where our therapeutic and life experience suggests some families can handle perceived crises successfully, while other, and more vulnerable ones cannot.

On the other hand, there are many situations where a recent occurrence threatens to devastate a family's ability to survive or meet its basic goals. These are events that would be devastating to any family's functioning, even the most resilient. They include a loss of job, a natural disaster, a death or serious illness, a parental separation and other similar events. Often such events occur quickly and unexpectedly. Their stress is usually traumatic. Often, family therapists treating the family in crisis have difficulty assessing the objective seriousness of crises. One reason is that we tend to ignore the seriousness of the stress and concentrate instead on the family pathology. It is important to assess the two separately. This is illustrated below, in a highly pathological family discussed at length:

Family Study 3.3. The Kellers

Rhea is a 44-year-old divorced mother of three. She is employed as a secretary. Her ex-husband lives on an opposite coast and provides no emotional and only sporadic financial support for the children. Rhea reports being hard-pressed financially, stressed at work, and somewhat depressed over the lack of a romantic relationship in her life. She describes herself as being very religious and the family's principal social life revolves around various activities of a large, nondenominational fundamentalist church "where we have real values."

Rhea presents to the local mental health clinic stating that her family is "in an unsolvable crisis." She has been referred by an assistant pastor who stated that the family "needs to be evaluated for mental health" (sic). Rhea sobs to the intake worker that her whole family "is out of control." Her daughter Sarah, 15, has recently expressed her desire to quit school the following year, as soon as she is legally able. Sarah's stated goal is to go out west to stay with her father. When told that she would not be allowed to do this, Sarah responded by telling her mother to "fuck off" and angrily left the house.

These sentiments are apparently reinforced by the children's father's mother, who maintains weekly contact with her grandchildren and provides them with occasional spending money.

Rhea's 12-year-old son, Kyle, is characterized as "the good child, my little helper. Without him this family would be lost." Kyle is very bright and does well in school. He is popular and successful in sports. Much of the routine family chores are delegated to him, a position his mother believes he relishes. Kyle, however, has told his school counselor that he is "tired of playing junior dad" at home and that he "want(s) to be like a normal kid."

The third child, Jason, "my baby doll," is 7 years old. Jason is seen by Rhea as being very emotional, but "special." His demeanor of "entitledness" is obvious in the first family interview. Rhea states that Jason is the "blessed child" since "he almost died at birth because my ex-husband hit me so many times when I was pregnant." According to Rhea, "the doctors think his nervous system didn't develop right and he's a little hyper. Sometimes he gets on my nerves. Then I smack him, like it says in the Bible to do. Sometimes I ignore him. He'll grow out of it." She also adds that "every time I think of him, I remember the way that evil man (her ex-husband) treated me."

Rhea states the immediate precipitant for contacting the mental health center was "my daughter's outrageous behavior. She's become simply uncontrollable. She listens to heavy metal music and just won't behave herself . . . Her room is a pigsty." However, Rhea states that she has considered counseling "for some time," but "I've just been too busy to do it, with the kids and all."

Family therapists of just about any orientation would immediately note numerous problems with Rhea's family: boundaries, coalitions, parentified children, psychodynamic projections, lack of consistent reinforced behavior, inappropriate punishment, poor parenting skills, and many other difficulties. Rhea presents to the clinic as being "completely overwhelmed . . . I can't function." And yet, despite family pathology and obvious external stress, deeper inquiry indicates that Rhea is performing relatively well. She is working a second job to augment the family coffers and is also attending night school to learn accounting. However, she *believes* her situation is out of control and this belief seems to influence the family's functioning.

PERCEPTUAL CRISES

Rhea's family illustrates that many crisis cases originate from parents who feel they have "had the last straw." A long series of gradual behaviors of various family members has often escalated. Usually, there is one salient precipitant that made participants declare "I've had enough!" Sometimes crises are provoked by a belief that an implicit family rule has been broken (Jackson, 1965). Subjectively, these crises are extremely severe and place great stress on the person in crisis as well as the entire family system. However, it is often difficult for the therapist to ascertain "Exactly why did you come in to treatment today?"

In evaluating this type of family crisis, the therapist often wonders to him/herself not only "What prompted you now?" but also "Why didn't they come see me years ago?" Invariably, when asked this question, the client will respond, "I never realized the problem was that bad." Often the sudden "insight" into the family problem's severity occurs only after intervention from other and more powerful social systems, such as the police or school officials.

This type of stress can be labelled as a perceptual stress. This name is appropriate for two reasons. First, this realization of family dysfunction is often a new belief, a new perception, or at least one that was rarely overtly voiced. Often there has been little immediate change in a family's function to provoke the stress. What has changed is the person's internal representation or perception of the situation. Quite frequently, this change comes about as a result of intervention from an outside social system.

Secondly, as we have seen in Rhea's case, there is usually a perception that the family is "out of control." Individuals feel simultaneously helpless and angry at their situation. They perceive their options to be limited in the face of the need for immediate action.

Perceptual stresses, then, are characterized by two attributes. One is the relatively new insight into the fact that there is indeed a family problem, despite signs of apparent long-standing difficulty. Second is the perception of personal and familial helplessness, frustration, anger, and the need for immediate action. This is illustrated in the rather graphic dialogue between a crisis worker and a distraught clinic "walk-in," an authoritarian middle-aged Marine sergeant.

Family Study 3.4. Sergeant Tallmeyer

Therapist: Now can you tell me please what brings you here?

C: (angrily) I just found out that my son is a homo.

Therapist: Gay?

C: You got it. (Hands wringing, and appearing very agitated)

Therapist: Yes, go on . . .

C: I mean . . . I mean, I don't know what to do . . . (resigned). I mean, like, he's 17 years old, and I get this call from the assistant principal saying, I have some bad news. I think your son is a queer.

Therapist: Hmm. He said that? Ah, just like that?

C: Yeah. I mean . . . Well, I think he used the word 'homosexual', but whatever . . . whatever . . . They found a letter he wrote to another boy in his . . . in the hall . . . in the locker or fallen out of the locker or something. And it described all kinds of . . . Oh, God, I'm going to be sick. It just disgusts me.

Therapist: You had no clue to your son's orientation–his sexual orientation?

C: Oh, of course not, I mean . . . I mean . . . I should have known earlier. Maybe I could have gotten him cured or something . . . And then they opened his locker and found a magazine with the letter. The principal said it had pictures of men together. Jesus Christ! I mean, what can I do? Is there any place I should take him to get him cured?

Therapist: We can talk about that in a few minutes. But right now, I'm curious. You had no idea until today?

C: No, I mean, yes . . . . goddamn it, I don't know. I mean, maybe, maybe I had a suspicion. I should have done something before. Maybe if I hadn't left him here with his mother when I went overseas . . . (head buried in hands). Jesus, my son a faggot. I'd rather him be dead . . . Why the fuck didn't I know?

Therapist: And you had no idea of his orientation until today?

C: Hell, I probably did. The clues were there. I'm a fucking idiot . . . That's me. An idiot. I mean the goddamn kid was 17 and he never dated, never bought any girlie magazines, never watched football. Never was like, a real man, you know . . . (crying). Hell, of course I knew. I'm a idiot. I thought, maybe hey, the kid's a little slow to develop it. I even took him to the doctor on base about that but you know how they are at _____. The doctor didn't say shit. "He's normal" they said.

Therapist: And right now you are feeling . . .

C: My only son and I could have stopped it . . . I've got to do something . . . I'm feeling like I got to do something. (Pause). I'm going to throw the little fucker out . . . That's it. Let his boyfriend take care of him. I don't want any little faggot sleeping in my house.

This explicit exchange illustrates many of the attributes of the perceptual stress. Following community pressure, the sergeant feels a sudden "denouement," followed by a helpless rage and a feeling of needing to act ("I've got to do something!"). He blames himself for not knowing, and then realizes "The clues were there." He feels guilt over not acting previously. He now feels he needs to act and rashly proposes a plan to force his underage son to leave home.

INSTRUMENTAL STRESS

These types of stressors contrast with another categorization: stressors which feature a sudden onset, generally with little chronicity and with an extreme disruption of personal and family functioning. The crisis interview below illustrates some of these features.

Family Study 3.5. The Hinsons

> *Therapist:* Now, what seems to be the problem?
>
> *Joan:* It's John's son.
>
> *John:* (interrupting) It's my son, Allen. He's 22. He's . . . well . . . we just found out he has AIDS.
>
> *Therapist:* Yes, go on.
>
> *John:* He came home for the holiday. We've not seen too much of each other since the divorce right before he went to college. And right after dinner, he tells us that he's got it. We're numb. I mean, I don't care who he sleeps with and that, but I just don't want him to die.
>
> *Joan:* I mean, we don't . . . (crying). We don't know what to do . . . We weren't close to him, not since John's divorce. But, it's like a death sentence, isn't it? Is there any hope?
>
> *Therapist:* Did he just test positive, or was he diagnosed for AIDS?
>
> *John:* Uh, I don't know. I don't know anything about it. I don't know what to do, who to turn to, you know? I mean, I could call Dr. _____, but it's a small town. I don't even know, I mean, if it's safe to have him around or should he be in the hospital or what?
>
> *Joan:* We want to do the right thing, but we have children at home. And, this is the first visit that Alan has made to us in a while and I . . . we just don't know. I mean, if there was some experimental treatment or someplace, maybe someplace he could go. I read that it is more contagious in the summer and some people believe mosquitoes can spread it.[1] We live by the woods, and I worry about my kids. Our kids.
>
> *John:* There's . . . it's something you want to just make go away . . . Our world has been, well, it sounds stupid, but turned upside down.

---

1. There is absolutely no evidence to support this once popular mistaken belief.

Therapist: Yes, I understand.

John: You just want it to go away for good . . . (crying).

Joan: We don't know what to do next. We don't have a clue about what we should do. Where do we go for help?

This family typifies many of the features found in a different kind of family crisis than that evoked by perceptual stressors. The family above is immediately devastated and unable to formulate a course of action. Their capacity to make basic decisions regarding family welfare is temporarily impaired. Their world has been "turned upside down," and they may even decide to permanently exclude one of their members from the family. Essentially, their ability to meet the material needs of family members may be threatened. Indeed, this type of stress that John and Joan Hinsom have encountered seems much more objectively serious than that of Sergeant Tallmeyer.

When we speak of the objective seriousness of a family's stress, we mean the capacity of a stressor to seriously impede or even permanently destroy family functioning. Usually this is associated with crises that threaten the ability to meet biological needs of the family, including family members' safety. Unemployment, accident, illness, sudden financial ruin or natural disaster are all stressors that can unexpectedly and suddenly damage or destroy the family's abilities to clothe and feed itself or to provide shelter for its members. We refer to these type of stressors as *instrumental* stressors and crises evoked by instrumental stressors as *instrumental crises*.

The ratio of perceptual versus instrumental crises that the family therapist encounters depends upon his or her setting. In private practice, the distribution of cases is almost always skewed highly towards perceptual crises. In community mental health agencies, there is probably less skew. It is not uncommon, for example, for individuals to present to such clinics after experiencing the death of a loved one or loss of the family home to a hurricane or fire. In emergency mental health clinics and emergency rooms, therapists are much more likely to find a bias towards the instrumental stress. Most clients will not go to an emergency room in desperation over a spouse or child's behavior. They will go, however, when they are suicidal about not having a job or being able to feed their children.

The categorization of perception vs. instrumentality of stressors and crises is clearly not binary, but instead exists on a continuum. At one end of the continuum, we have events that could, in optimal situations, pose little disruption to family functioning. Yet they are often perceived as highly stressful by the family and may evoke a crisis. At the other end, we have events that clearly do pose serious instrumental threats of disruption of family tasks regardless of family strengths and resources.

Crises may also occupy a "middle ground" position regarding instrumentality and perceptuality. Or they may have features of both extremes. This can occur when individuals who are prone to perceptual crises encounter an instrumental stress that threatens to permanently destroy their family system capacity for adaptation and goal attainment.

Family pathology may or may not be serious in cases of instrumental crises. The case below is an "instrumental" stress and subsequent crisis with a family that is clearly highly pathological. (The reader may wish to note all the potential pathological features this narrative includes).

Family Study 3.6. The McNaultons

Jennifer McNaulton, age 14, placed a call to the local mental health center regarding her father and stepmother. Mr. Joe McNaulton, 43, found out from his mother that his brother, John, 37, has been having an affair with Joe's current wife (Jennifer's stepmother). Joe, a recovering alcoholic with several years of sobriety, has begun drinking again and, according to Jennifer, "talking about ending himself."

Joe openly tells the therapist on the phone that "I plan to sit here and drink myself to death unless I run across that bitch and maybe I'll take her with me." At this time, he is well on his way to inebriation.

Jennifer states that her stepmother, who works for Joe's brother John as a marketing representative, is due home from a business trip the following morning.

Joe and John's mother, Rita, 64, is contacted and says that

she is "glad to state my side of the story." She claims that "these boys have been behaving like this all their lives. Joe stole John's first wife, so I guess they're just evening it out a little." She states that she is not particularly worried about Joe's drinking because "he goes on and off the wagon all the time." She is more concerned, however, with John's increasing cocaine habit that he can no longer hide and the fact that John has been physically assaultive to his children. However, she admonishes the emergency worker not to fret, explaining that the men's father, Robert, is out of town on a business trip and "I suspect Bob will straighten those two boys out when he gets back. He usually does. A good talking to will solve their problems."

PERCEPTUAL CRISES AND TREATMENT RESISTANCE: AN EMPIRICAL STUDY

McCown and Johnson (1991) investigated the occurrence and severity of perceptual and instrumental crises in treatment resistant, high risk, and crisis-prone families, and in families without a history of either treatment resistance or crises. (The former group of families were operationally defined as "dysfunctional families," while the latter group were labeled as "functional." However, these are simply labels based on comparisons. The terms do not imply that the latter group of families was "normal" or well functioning.) The authors had therapists rate the presenting problems of 147 families at the time of clinical intake, following the families' first therapy sessions. Families were rated on an eleven-point scale designed to measure the continuum of stress instrumentality. Higher ratings were associated with presenting problems that were more instrumental. Ratings were made prospectively, with categorizations of families based on their future treatment termination or crisis-proneness.

One of the hypotheses advanced by the authors was that treatment resistant families would be more likely to present with instrumental problems, while crisis-prone families would be more likely to present to treatment with perceptual problems. This hypothesis was only partially supported. All three types of "dysfunctional" families studied had lower instrumental ratings than "functional" families. In other words, these three family types were significantly more likely to seek family treatment for perceptual, rather than instrumental problems. However, contrary to the initial prediction, there were no between group differences for these three family types.

These findings were based on the therapists' ratings at the time of intake. Ratings taken three weeks later correlated highly A with the therapists' initial ratings. This suggests that therapists were consistent regarding their assessment of instrumentality of presenting problems.

The same families, on the other hand, rated their own problems quite differently than their therapists. Family ratings were obtained from the person in the family system who made the initial contact for therapy services. Problems were rated on an eleven-point Likert-type scale once a week for three weeks. Since no scale for client ratings of instrumentality has been constructed two alternate variables were rated: "How much can you and your family control the problems you are having?" and "How disruptive are your current problems to your family?" These variables were chosen because a previous factor analytic study indicated that the instrumentality/perceptuality continuum included these two orthogonal dimensions.

All three dysfunctional family groups rated their presenting problems as highly uncontrollable (mean = 8.9, sd = 2.3), compared with normal families (mean = 6.2, sd = 4.9). Ratings of problem controllability remained relatively constant across the three sessions ($r = .72$). However, ratings of family disruption varied significantly between dysfunctional groups. On all three of the ratings, crisis-prone families evaluated their presenting problem as highly uncontrollable and disruptive. The ratings of disruptiveness correlated .86 across sessions one and three. High risk families were less consistent in their rates of disruptiveness across the three sessions ($r = .44$). Among treatment resistant families, there was only a low correlation between ratings for disruptiveness between the first and third week ($r = .22$).

These findings have a number of implications for therapeutic intervention. Treatment resistant, high risk, and crisis-prone families are more likely to receive services following a perceptual crisis than families who do not meet these criteria. Each of these family types are also likely to view their presenting problems as out of their control. However, treatment resistant and to a lesser extent, crisis-prone families quickly "habituate" to the seriousness of their presenting difficulty. While they maintain consistency in their belief that their problems are outside of their control, they quickly assume their problems are less serious. This data suggests that one of the reasons treatment resistant families drop out of therapy quickly, is that they adapt to the capacity of their presenting problem to disrupt their systems. What causes this adaptation? Although more research is clearly needed, we suggest that resistant and high risk families have more effective homeostatic mechanisms than crisis-prone and "functional" families. These homeostatic mechanisms apparently do not act to boost the subjective feelings of controllability of the crisis. Instead, they serve to convince the family that the impact of their presenting problem on their family system is trivial, and that the problem, while outside of their control, is not important.

Later chapters will address this point further, emphasizing the large number of dysfunctionality of coping styles usually associated with the treatment resistant family. We will argue that an abundance of *dysfunctional* coping styles is one of the reasons that resistant families have a more rapid return to homeostasis following a family crisis and subsequently disregard the need to make lasting changes. However, regardless of the etiology of this habituation, we maintain that specific treatment implications are suggested from the above findings. These are summarized below:

1. A prime goal for any family suspected of being treatment resistant, high risk, or crisis-prone should be to reduce the amount of stress in the system. This is necessary because such systems typically have excessive–often extraordinary–levels of current systemic tension. Below, we will address an additional theoretical reason for controlling stress levels in families.

2. Therapy with resistant, high risk and crisis-prone families should also strive to reduce the subjective feelings of uncontrollability regarding crises. Additional rationale and examples of controlling the perception of familial stress will also be addressed below.

3. Finally, for treatment resistant and high risk families (but not

for crisis-prone families), therapy should reiterate the potential disruptiveness of the problem at hand. This reiteration may be too disruptive for crisis-prone families, adding unnecessarily to the stress level. However, it may be vital for families who are likely to terminate treatment prematurely. Such reiteration may help convince these families that their problems are serious and worthy of sustained attention and effort.

FAMILIAL DIFFERENCES IN STRESS COPING

Why do some families seem able to resist extremely pernicious instrumental stressors, while other families are devastated by routine life transitions? This is a complex question, indeed. With the number of potential factors that can be seen to be related to coping with stressors, it is not surprising that a large body of literature has accumulated regarding models of stress and family functioning. Empirical approaches to family stress theory began in earnest during the Depression of the 1930s. Angell (1936) studied the stressor of the loss of family income from the Great Depression. Based on careful observation he asserted two major determinants of a family's reaction to catastrophic loss of wages. These were: (1) the degree of familial integration, or interdependence and mutual interest, and (2) the degree of adaptability, or flexibility, especially in decision making. Families optimally poised to handle stressors were the "plastic" families, those in which roles were interchangeable.

Cavan and Ranck (1938) performed one of the earliest longitudinal studies of family adaptation to stressors. Their work emphasized that well-organized families had a maximal chance of adapting to the stressors of sudden poverty. This contrasted with disorganized families, or families that had poor previous methods of meeting needs. Needless to say, the stress of unemployment exacerbated the difficulties of the disorganized family.

Koos (1946) studied the effects of chronic daily stressors on family functioning. These included the effects of chronic poverty on the ability of slum residents to effectively meet their environmental demands. By present standards of social science, Koos methods were somewhat subjective. However, Koos was able to demonstrate that chronic stressors impeded a family's ability to effectively cope with environmental demands. He also believed that industrial society was responsible for some of the inability of the family to weather stress. He made an eloquent plea for societal intervention to reduce disintegration of the family.

Hill (1949) was the most important family stress theorist of this, or perhaps any, period. Hill studied the effect of the stressor of separation due to World War II on families. He postulated that a family's ability to cope with stress was a function of integration, or coherence and adaptability or flexibility. Ten factors contributed to both desirable traits. These included:

1. Prior history of successfully dealing with crisis;
2. Predominance of nonmaterialistic family goals;
3. Flexibility and willingness to shift traditional roles if necessary;
4. Acceptance of responsibility of duties by all family members;
5. Willingness to sacrifice personal gains for the interests of the family;
6. Pride in the family and in ancestors;
7. The presence of strong emotional interdependence;
8. High participation by all family members in the family process;
9. Egalitarian family control and decision making; and
10. Strong affectional ties between family members including those between parents.

Later, Hill incorporated many of these into the popular model discussed below.

HILL'S ABC X MODEL OF FAMILY RESILIENCY

In response to the needs of social work clinicians who labored with crisis-prone and multi-problematic families, Hill presented his four factor framework for the effects of stress on family functioning. Hill's theory states that familial functioning following a crisis (which he labelled as "Variable X") is related to the strength of the environmental stressor ("A"), as modified by the family's resources ("B") and the family's collective psychological stress resilience ("C"). Families with fewer resources, such as social support, community integration, friends and relatives in the community, and with a greater sense of alienation from their neighbors are said to be at higher risk following extraordinary stressors. Family resilience includes psychological hardiness, acceptance of difficulties, positive appraisals of problems, and religious faith. Most models of family robustness that are presently in the literature are variants of Hill's (1949) ABC-X model. However, subsequent theorization has expanded this model considerably. Additional variables associated with family robustness to stressors have also been specified, most notably by McCubbin's prolific group. Family vulnerability ("V") is the family's level of previous stress, in part determined by external factors, and in part by normative internal demands (e.g., puberty of a child, birth of a new child, etc.). Vulnerability potentiates effects of traumatic stress. Family Typologies ("T") are defined as a set of basic attributes about the family system which characterizes and explains how the family typically behaves. Families that typically respond to crises in a balanced fashion are better able to cope with stress.

According to the Hill/McCubbin tradition, the absence of normal factors that would work to attenuate family stressors places a family at risk to be damaged by the stress. These numerous factors act as buffers to mediate the noxious effects of the stressor and perhaps also to return families to homeostasis following stress. Families with more positive factors are said to possess a degree of stress resistance. Families with less of these positive buffers are more prone to the effects of stressors and probably return less quickly to set point following stress.

THE HILL/McCUBBIN MODEL
AND TREATMENT RESISTANCE:
AN EMPIRICAL STUDY

McCown and Johnson (1992c) examined several variables of the Hill/McCubbin model in an effort to determine their relevance to treatment resistance. They attempted to ascertain which of these variables could discriminate between "functional" families receiving family therapy and "dysfunctional" families, namely those that were treatment resistant, high risk, or crisis-prone. As predicted, and in general support of the Hill/McCubbin model, each variable had a small to moderate discriminative ability. The most significant discriminator between "functional" and "dysfunctional" families was, somewhat surprisingly, the newest variable added to the McCubbin model, "PSC" or the degree to which families attempt to problem solve or cope as a unit. Perhaps this shouldn't be surprising. Many theorists (e.g., Haley, 1976) have commented that family pathology is causally linked to inabilities to problem solve successfully.

All three types of "dysfunctional" families also had elevated levels of life stressors, compared with "functional" families receiving treatment. This suggests–not surprisingly–that higher amounts of family stress are associated with more pathological functioning. These findings are a replication of our study discussed earlier.

McCown and Johnson sought to determine whether the Hill/McCubbin variables could discriminate among types of "dysfunctional" families. The variables did less well in discriminating between families as crisis-prone systems, high risk, or treatment resistant. An analysis of variance indicated minor differences between crisis-prone and treatment resistant families, but not between either of these two groups and high risk families. Somewhat unexpectedly, treatment resistant families were found to have greater resources (Variable C), including religious faith. On the basis of the Hill/McCubbin model, treatment resistant families appeared to be slightly less pathological than crisis-prone systems. While the clinician who answers the repetitive call from the crisis-prone family may disagree, we believe that these findings illustrate the inability of the model to adequately address the reasons for treatment resistance.

Other variables that we measured, however, we predicted categorization of crisis-proneness, high risk functioning, or treatment resistance. McCown and Johnson asked family spokespersons (Oster & Caro, 1990) to complete a Likert-type scale measuring satisfaction with existing levels of (a) community (b) social and (c) familial supports. Ratings were obtained at the first and third weeks of treatment. Families that terminated treatment by this date were reassessed by telephone.

Results revealed that resistant families had a relatively high level of satisfaction with their current levels of all three types of supports. High risk families had a moderate satisfaction with support levels, while crisis-prone families reported a lower overall level of satisfaction for these three variables.

Regarding the stability of ratings, satisfaction with support remained relatively constant over a three week period for crisis-prone (.67) and resistant families (.78). However, the ratings by high risk families varied considerably, and although positive, were low (.11).

In other words, treatment resistant families are consistently happy with their levels of community, social, and family supports. Crisis-prone families are consistently unhappy with these supports. High risk families are somewhat dissatisfied, yet ambivalent and tend to change their minds regarding their satisfaction.

The implications of these findings for family therapy of resistant and crisis-prone families are important. Treatment resistant families are happier with their supports than other families. Perhaps it is this happiness that encourages them to discount the seriousness of their presenting problem, as seen in the study by McCown and Johnson (1991). As three decades of research on the Hill/McCubbin model suggest, support variables buffer the effects of crises. If resistant families perceive their supports to be adequate, they are unlikely to seek or want profit from family therapeutic intervention.

On the other hand, crisis-prone families are very unhappy with their levels of support. Perhaps one of the reasons they are frequently in a crisis modality is that they have or perceive that they have insufficient supports to mediate the stresses of life. We would expect these families to remain in therapy, albeit a rocky course. This is precisely what happens.

Finally, high risk families are ambivalent about their systemic supports. Their evaluations change substantially, even in a three-week period. This may be due to the fact that their resources fluctuate or these families perceive their resources as unstable. This unstable source of community and family buffers causes the cycle of treatment resistance, termination, and subsequent new crisis.

As the study of McCown and Johnson (1991) reported earlier in the chapter, the present study has treatment implications for resistant, high risk, and crisis-prone families. These are summarized below:

1. Treatment resistant, high risk, and crisis-prone families can all benefit from interventions designed to enhance their capacity to solve problems together.

2. Interventions designed *solely* to boost the social or familial supports of resistant families may be ineffective, inasmuch as these families are typically happy with their current levels of support. Such interventions should probably be accompanied by an effort on the part of the therapist to weaken existing perceptions of the adequacies of present support levels. On the other hand, such interventions may be very effective for crisis-prone families. High risk families are ambivalent about support and could benefit from interventions designed to provide them with better and more consistent supports.

FAMILY STRESS AND OPPONENT PROCESSES

We have stated that one of our aims for reducing resistance is to diminish the family's level of systemic stress. The reason for this is not self-evident. Some family therapists may even feel somewhat uncomfortable with our emphasis on lessening tension in the resistant family system. Other schools of family therapy often act in reverse, attempting to enact change by increasing the tension in the system. As we have said previously, these methods of stress induction may be countertherapeutic in the resistant family, since early termination may occur simultaneously with the destabilization. However, we have another, perhaps more technical and speculative reason for trying to decrease the negative systemic forces in the resistant family.

Systemic response to stress is nonlinear and somewhat random. However, we believe that homeostatic family mechanisms follow an *opponent process*. The opponent-process theory of acquired motivation represents an extension of learning theory to a wide variety of powerfully motivated behaviors in humans and animals (Solomon & Corbit, 1974; Solomon, 1980). These include imprinting behavior of ducklings to mother objects, distress calls in young birds, and, in humans, romantic love and marathon running. Although the theory is primarily involved in explaining learning, it has application to a variety of nonlinear systemic behaviors.

The opponent process theory states that homeostasis (labeled the "B" state) occurs in response to intense stimulation of any type (labeled the "A" state). Each B state is a slow forming mirror image of the activation that caused it. Initially, homeostasis is calibrated fairly exactly with the degree of intensity of stimulation. Intense stimuli trigger intense but slower acting homeostatic compensators, while milder stimuli cause a much more moderate opponent response.

However, according to the opponent process theory, (Solomon, 1980) *repeated exposure* to the A state of any stimulus changes the parameters of its opponent B state. The opponent state becomes increasingly longer, reduced in latency, and greater in opponent intensity. An example from substance abuse is useful. The first phase of substance usage–that experienced by new users–is characterized by a sluggish and shallow opponent state, resulting in a primary stimulus–namely, the drug–producing a long effect. The second phase, habituation, is characterized by a B state that increases in intensity, duration and frequency of onset so that it cancels out some of the hedonic properties of the initial A state. This A/B balance is theorized to be the mechanism behind habituation, or decreased capacity of the drug user to experience a "high."

Stimulus tolerance occurs when the A and B states are of approximate equal duration. In this situation the use of a substance triggers both its primary affective state and its opponent state simultaneously. This is true because repeated exposure to an A state results in earlier onset of the opponent B mechanism. Eventually, the net hedonic effect is zero.

Exposure past the point of tolerance to any hedonically intense stimulus results in an even greater B state, in which case the hedonic value (A-B) is *negative*. Thus, stimulus administration causes more appetitively opponent responses than the initial stimulus A state. Solomon (1980) has suggested that this process is the explanation of the process of drug craving. Since its removal is best accomplished by the physiological antithesis–namely the A state–an individual will seek to readminister the A state stimulus to gain escape from the noxious B state. This has the effect of increasing the addiction, establishing the vicious cycle that characterizes addiction.

We believe that stress in families follows an opponent process. Treatment resistant families are much like the recovering heroin abuser who experience craving after just one slip. Such families encounter hypersensitized compensatory mechanisms in response to systemic stresses. Any stress in the family system causes an inappropriately large homeostatic opponent process. This excessive homeostasis is associated with resistance. Therefore, we seek to minimize resistance by reducing the overall level of family stress as much as is possible.

Admittedly, we have little data at this point to support this position. Such data requires a complex longitudinal study with literally thousands of observations, and this work is in progress. At this time, however, our clinical experience strongly suggests that reducing family stress reduces subsequent resistance. We find the opponent process model the most cogent explanation for this clinical phenomena. Therefore, unless there are other substantial clinical implications, we work rapidly to reduce the family tension with systems that might be resistant.

This rather technical discussion can be clarified with two simple visual illustrations. Figure 3.1 and 3.2 depict the hypothetical results of different levels of stress on a single family system. In Figure 3.1, a high level of stress generates a disproportionately deeper homeostatic response (a large B state). Higher levels of stress encourage greater systemic forces acting in opposition to neutralize the stress. This results in greater resistance to change and the family becomes more entrenched in its behavior.

Figure 3.2 represents the effects of a lower level of stress on the same family. Note that much less homeostasis is encountered following the lower stress level. Reduced family stress generates a B state of less intensity. There is much less likelihood of generating excessive family resistance in this situation. The system remains more flexible to change and therapeutic intervention.

The opponent process theory of family stress explains another

FIGURE 3.1. Opponent Response to Elevated Stress

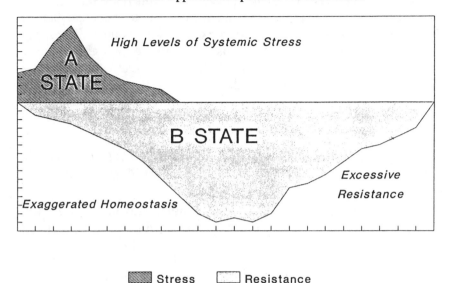

FIGURE 3.2. Opponent Response to Reduced Stress

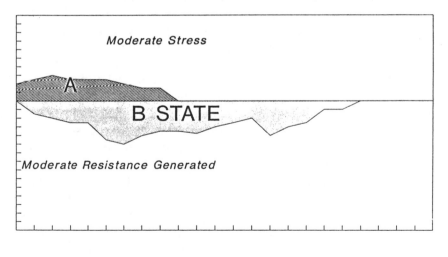

reason why we perform crisis intervention with resistant families. We must act quickly because we need to dissipate the stress before it reaches levels where it can cause excessive resistance. The rapid techniques of crisis intervention discussed in the next chapter give us a potent tool for reducing the likelihood of treatment failure by quickly reducing pressures on the family system to overcompensate.

THE PERCEPTION OF STRESS AS A CRITICAL VARIABLE IN CRISIS-PRONENESS AND TREATMENT RESISTANCE

Because of opponent processes and other reasons it is usually critical to reduce the overall stress level in the resistant family's system. The Hill/McCubbin model emphasizes that one of the major buffering factors regarding stress is family perception of the stressor. Our family studies thus far reiterate that crises occur when perceptions suddenly change. When family stress is perceived as uncontrollable, people feel they have reached the "last straw." A perceptual crisis often ensues. Perceptions, to a large degree, determine when stress produces a crisis.

The studies of stressors by Lazarus and his colleagues (e.g., Lazarus, 1966; Lazarus, 1984; Lazarus & Folkman, 1984) suggest that it is not a particular event per se that is stressful, but instead is the individual's interpretation or cognition associated with the event. Lazarus and Folkman (1984), for example, have supplied data from several interesting experiments demonstrating that cognition precedes the experience of stressors as being stressful. They conclude that in order for an event to be stressful, it must first be perceived as such.

Behavioral scientists have increasingly focused on a related component of the subjective assessment of stress, namely its capacity to be controlled. A consistent literature has emerged indicating that uncontrollable stress is much more aversive than controllable stressors (Lazarus & Folkman, 1984). Consequently, a number of coping procedures have been developed to facilitate cognitive control of stress. The goal of these coping procedures is to provide the client with a positive experience of stress controllability. When the client develops a history of positive control, he or she is said to acquire a stress inoculation.

Conversely, a history of exposure to uncontrollable stress may interfere with the future perception of stress controllability. When humans or other animals have a history of being exposed to uncontrollable environmental stressors, they show future deficits in escaping from reducible stress situations. They also show cognitive and behavioral changes that strikingly parallel those seen in depression. These changes in mammals include deficits in problem solving, reduced libido, reduced capacity to learn new material, attention problems, reduced eating and weight loss. This well-known phenomenon is called "learned helplessness" and was advanced by Seligman and Maier (1967) to account for their finding that an organism's perception of environmental contingencies significantly affects behavior. Maier and Seligman (1976) have suggested that learned helplessness can be broken down into three primary components: motivational, cognitive, and emotional. While much of the learned helplessness research has been conducted with animals, studies using human subjects have yielded very similar findings.

The effects of a familial history of uncontrollable stressors upon subsequent family helplessness is a comparatively new area of research that warrants more attention. Our belief is that many of the problems in urban communities, such as violence, substance abuse, and unemployment are the result of learned helplessness, especially regarding family behavior. Clearly, more research is needed regarding this issue. The effects of learned helplessness on family functioning are commonly encountered in the clinic, as the family study below indicates. Note that the client makes several erroneous attributions regarding the causes of her misfortunes.

Family Study 3.7. The Williamsons

Susan Williamson, a 35-year-old divorced woman, was referred to family therapy by the principal of her 7-year-old daughter, Danielle. Danielle, a charming and precocious child was thought to be somewhat hyperactive by her classroom teacher. A full neurological work-up failed to reveal either physical or behavioral abnormalities outside of the classroom.

Susan was a secretary of a large corporation that had just laid off some of its workers. Susan suspected that she might be next. Although perfectionistic and receiving excellent job performance reviews, she blamed the possibility of her layoff on her own incompetence. "I always get fired," she said mournfully. "All my life I can't do anything right."

Susan's therapist found her a very difficult client to work with. Susan would say little, almost nothing if she could help it. Occasionally she would smile meekly or laugh a few seconds too late. She also seemed preoccupied and socially awkward. At first, the therapist suspected a thought disorder, until this was ruled out by psychological testing. The therapist remained uncomfortable and perplexed.

During the second session, it became apparent that Susan desperately needed behavior-oriented parenting skills. Although she was compliant regarding their instruction, Susan seemed utterly incapable of performing at home anything she had learned in the therapy sessions. The therapist surmised that she tried, but simply gave up when events were slightly unpredictable or aversive. For example, when trying to administer a "Time Out" procedure to the recalcitrant Danielle, she stopped abruptly because "Danielle said she hated me and I didn't know what to do next. We didn't cover that one last week (in the session)."

Although Susan denied that she was depressed (and in fact had few vegetative signs) she appeared to give up easily and tire frequently. When questioned about this she stated that she had never been "much of a trier. I guess I'm afraid to stick to things."

After the fifth session, Susan was laid off from her job, along with the 40 other employees of her entire section. Her response was to blame herself, despite the fact that her boss and his boss had all been fired as well. Although a coworker had a "sure lead" at another local firm, Susan never applied for the position. She was extremely reluctant to file for unemployment compensation, and seemed anxious at the thought of doing so.

Susan terminated therapy after a few more sessions. She

sheepishly stated that her boyfriend didn't want her to go to therapy and he would get mad at her if she continued to do so. Several months later, Susan returned unscheduled to the agency and in extreme crisis. She was threatening suicide in the waiting room and had already scratched her wrist. She was also inebriated. She demanded to speak with her former therapist. She then told him that she had just discovered that her boyfriend had been molesting her daughter for the past two years. The police had been notified about this by Susan's ex-husband, who became suspicious about his daughter's sexual knowledge. The court was about to remove Danielle from the home and the DA would possibly press charges against her.

At that point Susan then admitted that her boyfriend had also been physically and sexually abusing her as well. Furthermore, her uncle had sexually molested her from the time she was nine until she was fifteen. Although she had a clear recollection of all of these events, she had never told her therapist of any of them because "I felt dirty and useless . . . and besides, someone as low as me deserves to be treated that way."

Based on the above discussion, we argue that systems like Susan's can eventually control the impact of stress on their system by changing their perceptions. Actual decrease in the objective stressors is but one, and perhaps the least important facet of this process. Psychological belief in controllability of the environmental stress is a second, and usually key component of crisis mastery. To help these systems we must convince the family that their stressors are controllable. This heightened sense of controllability will reduce future crisis-proneness.

The dilemma that practitioners face working with systems like Susan's is in modeling both stress controllability and realism. Not all stresses can or should be controlled. Furthermore, excessive confidence regarding the controllability of stressors often results in the characteristic *la belle indifference* to dysfunctionality that is repeatedly encountered in the resistant family. To reduce resistance we must convince the family that the stresses it faces are manageable, but also *potentially* disruptive and harmful. Overconfidence in stress coping is associated with treatment resistance, while inconsistent appraisal of stress or coping results in the cycle of treatment resistance and crisis-proneness characteristic of the high risk family. Families in crisis need to hear two messages: realistic controllability and consistency.

Therefore, our goal with families in crisis is to convince them that their problems are indeed serious, but also potentially manageable. Their problems are solvable as long *as they maintain efforts to solve them*. In other words, the onus of success or failure in therapy, as well as other endeavors in life, is up to the family. We emphasize that the family's efforts must be *consistent*, even when the symptoms disappear and the crisis is apparently allayed. This is because resistant families vacillate regarding their assessment of how serious they believe their crises actually are. The process of encouraging families to act optimistically and yet consistently is what we call family empowerment and is one of the cornerstones of our intervention with the resistant family.

Family empowerment is a process. One way it occurs is through successful crisis intervention. When the family solves its present crisis it becomes more convinced that its other difficulties are manageable. The effort expended in this crisis resolution becomes an invaluable lesson in teaching the family that its efforts do matter and in defeating family learned helplessness. Through successful crisis resolution future resistance is gradually diminished and change becomes possible. This is yet another reason why we advocate crisis intervention with resistant families.

Chapter Four

Family-Oriented Crisis Intervention

AN OVERVIEW TO A NEW METHOD
OF DEFEATING RESISTANCE

There are many reasons why crisis intervention is useful and necessary with resistant family systems. In Chapter One we presented data suggesting that treatment resistant families often received therapy primarily during or immediately following a crisis. Furthermore, we showed that resistant families are frequently crisis-prone, increasing the likelihood they will receive services in response to an actual or perceived emergency. In Chapter Three we suggested that rapid reduction in family stress can potentially reduce family resistance. Because of these and other factors, we advocate a method of family intervention with potentially resistant families that has borrowed many of its methods from family-oriented crisis intervention approaches. This chapter will discuss general techniques of family crisis intervention, emphasizing particular goals with resistant families.

An advantage to the crisis-oriented approach lies in its applicability to the early stages of therapy for most family problems. This is important inasmuch as presence or degree of family resistance is often unknown until the family abruptly terminates or fails to follow through with therapeutic recommendations. Therefore, we generally assume that any system we are interviewing for the first time has the potential to be treatment resistant and terminate prematurely. The crisis-oriented intervention strategies we advocate allow the therapist to meet the twin goals that he or she has done all that is possible to encourage compliance as well as empower the family to help itself in the event they abruptly terminate treatment.

Another practical advantage of the crisis intervention approach to the treatment of resistant families is that it is highly flexible. Therapists can initiate intervention with crisis related techniques, but retain the flexibility to change intervention strategies if such techniques are not appropriate to the family's presenting problem. Initial use of crisis techniques avoids locking the therapist into a single modality or a premature manner of facilitating change. Such interventions allow the therapist to defuse the family tension and simultaneously collect much needed information. Or, if the therapist makes an error (a frequent occurrence with resistant systems), the error can be more easily corrected.

Crisis intervention also allows the therapist maximum freedom to meet the family's unique needs. As we have learned from dynamical systems theory, the interaction of complex systems is variable and typically unpredictable. It is impossible to have a single agenda or treatment strategy that can meet all of the potential needs of resistant families during the initial interview. This is especially true during the first therapy session when the ground rules of therapy are less explicit. Crisis intervention allows the therapist the flexibility to do whatever is necessary to assist the family, without concerns regarding therapist roles or expectations. This can be critical when families present with a severe instrumental crisis.

A crisis intervention approach offers another useful and pragmatic benefit for the family therapist working with resistant families. This technique allows the therapist to observe the manner in which the system responds to change. For example, do family members communicate better when tension in the family is decreased? When suicidal ideation of the IP dissipates, do other family members become symptomatic? In traditional family or individual treatment, therapists are often too busy or involved to notice unexpected changes in the system. However, crisis intervention is similar to a laboratory experiment. That is, the opportunity to observe and test various hypotheses regarding family dynamics, functioning, and reaction to stress is presented.

Still another boon of crisis intervention techniques is that they provide a "hands on" approach with immediate results. The emphasis on direct, active, and focused problem solving is usually a welcome change for families who have previously failed in more prolonged treatments. The resistant system's belief that change is possible is enhanced through the process of efficient problem solving. Often, this is a useful antidote to a history of treatment resistance and crisis-proneness. Similarly, rapid and efficient problem solving may circumvent homeostatic mechanisms that typically impede family change. Rapid change also allows for an abrupt shift in family self-organization (Chamberlain, 1991) that makes the homeostatic resistance of difficult systems less problematic.

This chapter will focus on the history and efficacy of family-oriented crisis intervention. We will then discuss some goals for family-oriented crisis intervention with potentially resistant systems, and useful models of family-oriented crisis intervention. We will then present our own model and interventions, with emphasis on empowerment and reducing dysfunctional family coping. Finally, we will highlight the differences between traditional crisis intervention and preventative intervention we advocate for resistant families.

FAMILY-ORIENTED CRISIS INTERVENTION: A BRIEF HISTORY

During the mid-1960s to the early 1980s many clinicians began to observe the value of family involvement during emergency psychiatric consultation or crisis intervention. Although the use of family-oriented crisis intervention is probably as old as the profession of social work, the first widespread use of the family in crisis intervention began in earnest in the late 1960s. Family Crisis Therapy (FCT) was a specific type of brief intervention pioneered by the group at the Family Treatment Unit of the Colorado Psychiatric Hospital (Langsley & Kaplan, 1968; Pittman, 1973). The model of FCT focused on identification and resolution of the stress-induced crisis. Crisis is resolved by the family making changes either to remove or adapt to the stress.

An evaluation of FCT suggests it is a highly effective program to reduce need for psychiatric hospitalization (Langsley, Pittman, Machotka, & Flomenhaft, 1968; Langlsey, Pittman, & Swank, 1969). In one study, three hundred patients were randomly assigned to either psychiatric hospitalization or to FCT. FCT patients were less likely to require hospitalization during a six-month follow-up. Additionally, FCT patients were returned to their usual roles about two-and-a-half times sooner than hospitalized patients. Although differences in rates of rehospitalization leveled out over longer periods time, FCT was at least a short-term and cost effective program to deter repeated hospitalization.

Subsequent literature has stressed the usefulness of employing family systems theory for crisis intervention (Buchanan & Chasnoff, 1986; Levy & McCown, 1983). Although much confusion remains regarding the role of families during crisis intervention (Worthington, 1987), the following trends have occurred in the crisis intervention and family therapy literature as well as in clinical practice.

THEORETICAL RATIONALE
FOR FAMILY CRISIS INTERVENTION

By the mid-1980s many family-oriented clinics were routinely handling crisis calls by insisting upon involvement of the client's family (Levy & McCown, 1983). There are a number of theoretical reasons family crisis intervention might prove more successful than interventions involving only one family member. Some of these reasons are reviewed briefly below.

The Family as Historians

One major use for family intervention during psychiatric emergencies is to establish a reliable client history. The client's view of his or her presenting problem during a crisis is not necessarily the view that others in the family share. A standard of community care for crisis intervention is that the client's history and presenting complaints be corroborated by other family members whenever possible (Newhill, 1989). The case presented below indicates how the family can be used to gather useful, and often essential, treatment information.

Case Study 4.1. The Kilroys

Mr. Kilroy called a hospital late one fall afternoon reporting that he felt suicidal. He stated that he had a history of seven psychiatric hospitalizations for depression and that he was "off my meds for a while." He was positive for suicidal ideation and vegetative signs of depression, but was vague regarding suicidal plan. He could give no reason for his feelings, only perseverating loosely that "My whole life has fallen apart and I'm to blame."

The clinician who conducted the telephone interview, a second year psychiatric resident, noted in the hospital contact log that the patient sounded like a "case of severe unipolar depression" who experienced "periodic endogenous exacerbation." The patient was told to come in immediately for an interview and that hospitalization might indeed be necessary.

At the insistence of the clinician, Mr. Kilroy was driven to the interview by his only available family member, a 16-year-old son named Harold. Surprisingly, Harold asked to be seen in private by the resident. Although the resident usually excluded family members from the initial crisis interview–he was psychoanalytically oriented and believed that family members might "contaminate" future treatment–he agreed to make an exception, based upon Harold's earnestness as well as his persistence. He told Harold he would talk with him after talking with the father. The resident then interviewed Mr. Kilroy, and began making plans for hospitalization.

Almost on his way out, the resident remembered his promise to Harold. He castigated himself for allowing valuable time to be spent with this young man when Mr. Kilroy's diagnostic formulation was so obvious. Besides, he found families troublesome and meddling, and contact with them usually upset the patient. Nevertheless, he had made a promise so he agreed to see the youth for five minutes.

Although Harold was inarticulate and nervous, his information was invaluable to the resident. Harold stated that he was "convinced that my Dad's–you know–problem, has something to do with the fact that he and Mom split up just today. My mom said she just couldn't stay with my dad unless he did something about his problem."

The Family as Symptom Managers

Family-oriented clinicians soon discovered the family to be not only helpful as historians, but also invaluable for managing client symptomatology. During the late 1970s and early 1980s, a number of innovative methods were employed by clinicians to encourage the family to manage client crises themselves, with a minimum of professional intervention. For example, the family might be asked to closely monitor a suicidal member. This might include fifteen minute "contact checks," removal of dangerous items, and daily "progress reports" to a crisis therapist. With a little experience, therapists began to realize that many previously "unmanageable" patients thought to invariably require hospitalization could be controlled in the less restrictive and certainly more economic environment of the client's home. Often, these procedures were employed by necessity, rather than for humanitarian reasons or value to the treatment process. For example, during the peak years of deinstitutionalization it was often extremely difficult for mental health workers to arrange hospital admission for indigent or lower middle-class families lacking mental health insurance. Deinstitutionalization, which started out primarily as a reform measure, soon became a way for state governments to slash budgetary requirements. Overcrowded state hospitals were curtailed in their services or closed, further overwhelming already strained existing inpatient resources. In some jurisdictions there were almost no emergency psychiatric beds available. Because of lack of resources, crisis workers became adept at encouraging the families of crisis patients to use their own resources to avert hospitalization.

During the last decade, this expertise was put to a greater test, as more and more families faced the specter of attempting to find treatment for a family member in the face of depleted resources. The plethora of private psychiatric hospitals that arose in recent years, especially under the Reagan era, had a seeming propensity for exhausting a family's psychiatric insurance coverage before pronouncing the patient "cured." When the patient "recycled," mental health workers in community agencies who were entrusted–or forced–to manage these now uninsured individuals had to develop novel methods of preventing suicide and psychiatric decompensation. Some of the heroes of this generation of therapists were the community-oriented family clinicians who struggled against bureaucratic indifference in an attempt to manage the serious emergencies that seemed to slip through the cracks and wind up on their caseloads.

Fortunately, some positive benefit accrued from this extreme effort. To many family-oriented clinicians, it became obvious that these "hospital deferment" interventions possessed positive therapeutic value. Families formerly characterized by little communication or indication of caring began to show respect, mutual tolerance, and even love toward each other. Hierarchies were reiterated and parents found they could indeed control their previously "uncontrollable" or "incorrigible" children. Therapists began to realize that in addition to management benefits, "pseudo hospitalizations" were having profound and usually positive effects on the family.

In our experience, *pseudohospitalization*, or intense family monitoring of an IP as an alternative to formal inpatient psychiatric hospitalization, possess a number of benefits. Specifically, it often strengthened the family hierarchy as parents began to behave more responsibly toward their children. In the process, parents accumulated more appropriate and effective parenting skills. Parents and children frequently demonstrated an increased vigor towards making progress in therapy, as if the pseudohospitalization experience had convinced them of the necessity for implementing changes themselves. Often, these families cease relying on an outside agent to "fix" their family member, but instead combine forces to heighten the probability they will not reexperience the crisis most recently and mutually managed. Perhaps most beneficially, intense family monitoring sometimes seems to promote positive interchange of emotion among family members whose normative standard for interaction formerly consisted largely of hostile interchange.

One of the most popular variations on the pseudohospitalization approach is "The Hospital-in-the-Home," where a ritualized procedure is employed to break the cycle of dependency upon inpatient hospitalization for crisis intervention. The basis of this intervention is to have the family recreate, as much as possible, the ambience and the inconvenience of a hospital experience while minimizing the rewards. Family members might organize in shifts as "staff" to monitor the "patient," who is often an adolescent with a history of multiple psychiatric hospitalizations. The "patient" would be restricted to his or her room, given a rigid schedule of "therapeutic" activities, "recreation time" (usually television watching with "staff"), and might even participate in "group therapy" with other family members.

An excellent example of the use of a hospital diversion technique for an adolescent is available in Landau-Stanton and Stanton (1985). This article should be required reading for anyone who attempts to manage a crisis in the home for any client family.

An experience with pseudohospitalization was attempted by the resident psychiatrist who interviewed Mr. Kilroy.

Case Study 4.1. The Kilroys (continued)

After initial discussion with Mr. Kilroy, the resident and Mr. Kilroy agreed that Mr. Kilroy was in need of and would seek voluntary hospitalization. However, the billing clerk reported to the resident that Mr. Kilroy's insurance did not cover inpatient care. In cases such as these, the hospital required that the patient pay a substantial amount of the fee upon admission, a condition that Mr. Kilroy was unable to do.

Since he had no insurance coverage, Mr. Kilroy would require hospitalization in a state facility, where the nearest available bed was 50 miles away. Furthermore, because Mr. Kilroy was a voluntary patient, he would have to secure his own transportation to the state hospital. The resident thought that this was too dangerous, as Mr. Kilroy might simply jump out of a moving vehicle or change his mind about hospitalization halfway into the trip. The only other option available to secure Mr. Kilroy a safe trip to a state bed was civil commitment, in which case the local magistrate would arrange for his hospitalization via local ambulance.

The situation was explained to Mr. Kilroy who agreed he had little choice but to be civilly committed. He requested, however, that his wife not be involved in the commitment because "she could use this against me if she decides to go through with the divorce." The resident acquiesced that this was an appropriate request. Because it was necessary to have a community member start the civil proceedings, the resident called a friend of the patient.

The friend, Barney, a longtime union buddy, shocked the resident. Barney insisted that Mr. Kilroy would "snap out of this in a day or two." Barney suggested that Mr. Kilroy should stay with him "until he can think about it." To the dismay of the resident (who feared a lawsuit if Mr. Kilroy attempted suicide), the patient decided that he was well enough to stay with Barney, or "maybe my cousin John down the street, at least until I can get my head straight." The resident then called John, the cousin, who reiterated his desire to keep Mr. Kilroy out of the hospital. "Sure, he can stay here. I've got plenty of room. What the hell else are family for?"

Both Barney and John agreed to monitor Mr. Kilroy twice a day for the next two weeks. In the meantime, Mr. Kilroy would receive antidepressant medication, dispensed daily from the pharmacy, to prevent the possibility of an overdose. Mr. Kilroy also agreed to avoid drinking or drug use during this period. He further agreed to tell John or Barney if he was planning suicide. All parties agreed to call the resident daily until Mr. Kilroy could be seen for regular therapy, which was not until the end of the week.

The resident found it was relatively easy to maintain Mr. Kilroy as an outpatient. Each person held up their end of the therapeutic contract. Although Mr. Kilroy's depression lingered for some time, an expensive and potentially stigmatizing hospitalization was avoided.

The Family as the Cause of the Crisis

During the late 1970s and 1980s progressive clinicians began to investigate the role of family processes in facilitating psychiatric crises. Interpersonal crises began to be viewed as but one (albeit, one of the more serious) aspect of a dysfunctional family system. Family therapists noted that rarely did symptoms such as alcoholism, depression, and even schizophrenia occur in a systemic vacuum (Framo, 1965). Instead, familial precipitants could clearly be identifiable in the histories of most crisis cases. Implicit or explicit family rules often seemed to govern the crisis-oriented behavior of family members, as well as other aspects of the family's life-style.

To the family therapist, the individual psychiatric crisis seemed to serve a familial function (Sugarman & Masheter, 1986). This was evident by its regularity, repetitiveness, and patterns observed in family activity and emotionality during and after the crisis. The function of the crisis was rarely understood by family members, or even by the numerous therapists who were usually involved with these families. However, longitudinal examination of these "crisis-prone" families indicated periodic phases of tranquility punctuated by predictable crises of some type and then a refractory "honeymoon period" of indeterminate, yet transitory duration. This cycle can be seen in exploration of additional details of the Kilroy family, below:

Case Study 4.1. The Kilroys (continued)

> The resident began seeing Mr. Kilroy for weekly psychotherapy. Although Mr. Kilroy was no longer suicidal, he remained seriously depressed. Numerous antidepressant combinations, including MAO inhibitors were tried, but to no avail. The resident voiced fears to his colleagues that by seeing the family in the initial interview he had "hopelessly contaminated the transference." After several weeks of unresponsiveness to treatment, the resident suggested to his supervisor that the patient might need to receive electroconvulsive therapy (ECT) on an inpatient basis.

> The supervisor, however, suggested that the resident might wish to begin by interviewing the entire family in the presence of Mr. Kilroy. Although the resident was puzzled by the suggestion, and even a little alarmed, he was also desperate. After receiving Mr. Kilroy's permission, the resident telephoned the wife's home and asked the entire family to come in for at least one session. Although Mrs. Kilroy was hostile to the idea that "I should help that son-of-a-bitch," she agreed to bring herself and her other two children, as well as Harold, to the next therapy session.

Despite initial acquiescence by Mrs. Kilroy, she was a "no-show" at the family meeting. All three children, however, attended the session. After interviewing the two other children living in the home, Janet, age 21, and Michael, age 19, the following facts emerged regarding Mr. Kilroy's depression and recent stress of apparently impending divorce:

1. This was the seventh time in 11 years Mr. Kilroy's wife had threatened to sue him for divorce.
2. Each incident followed confrontation by the wife regarding the patient's numerous extramarital affairs.
3. Confrontation was habitually followed by the wife's binge drinking, which invariably resulted in mutual domestic violence and the patient's expulsion from the home, sometimes by court order and sometimes at gunpoint by the wife's brothers.
4. At this point in the crisis cycle, Mr. Kilroy would seek psychiatric hospitalization, usually at the Veterans Affairs hospital.
5. During hospitalization, Mrs. Kilroy would usually refuse to visit her husband. However, the children would give her frequent reports regarding his status and mood. During this period, Mrs. Kilroy would almost always drink excessively, stating she needed alcohol to cope with her separation.
6. Mr. Kilroy's mental status would continue to deteriorate while his wife was drinking. Even electroconvulsive treatments (ECT), a powerful therapeutic tool, did little to interrupt his depression.
7. Usually, after the ECT regimen, Mrs. Kilroy would begin to feel guilty. She would then sober up and forgive her husband. In a few days, she would begin calling him on the telephone and his spirits would lift appreciably.
8. Invariably, Mr. Kilroy would sign out against medical advice (AMA), claiming that the ECT's had obliterated his memory not only for the hospitalization, but for the other women in his life.
9. Several months later, the cycle would renew. Mr. Kilroy

was never compliant with outpatient treatment for more than a few sessions following his hospitalization.

The Kilroy case highlights the importance of realizing the manner in which family factors dynamically interact to facilitate and precipitate psychiatric crises. This is not to say that other biopsychosocial factors are irrelevant in these or similar cases. For example, there was a history of maternal depression in Mr. Kilroy's family, with his mother and both of his maternal grandparents diagnosed as having "involutional melancholia." Similarly, Mrs. Kilroy's father had a history of episodic excessive drinking, usually prompted by stress. Regardless, we are forced to ask, as did the astute resident who treated the case, "Why do we have these symptoms *now*? Why not last week or month instead of today?" Often, viewing the timing of the symptom as adaptive will highlight treatment potentialities.

Case Study 4.1. The Kilroys (continued)

Upon realization of this "crisis pattern," the resident again requested Mrs. Kilroy to be seen in treatment with her husband. When contacted via telephone, Mrs. Kilroy was surprisingly pleasant, although she was clearly inebriated. Unexpectedly, she apologized for her absence from the previous session and also agreed to contact her husband. Within the next day both spouses agreed to the need for continued outpatient family treatment.

Under supervision the resident employed a structural/strategic framework for his interventions. His goal was to set about convincing each member of the couple that they were making "heroic sacrifices," such as suicidal ideation and binge drinking, in order to save their marriage. Both Mr. and Mrs. Kilroy resonated to this interpretation, and agreed that neither really wanted divorce. Tearfully, they forgave each other and agreed to a trial reconciliation.

By the second session, Mrs. Kilroy had stopped drinking completely. She had been sober for five days with no signs of withdrawal. Mr. Kilroy's depression had significantly lifted, largely in response to his wife's agreement to reunite.

Thinking strategically, the resident then explained to them that a "side effect" of their efforts to keep their marriage together had been the frequent problems with alcohol that Mrs. Kilroy had encountered, as well as the numerous bouts of depression that plagued Mr. Kilroy. In order to reduce their guilt regarding their lengthy history of dysfunctional symptoms, the resident also stressed that the etiologies of these diseases were primarily biological. He mentioned that their frequent use of the symptoms to preserve their marriage had caused the symptoms to "get out of hand, almost like when you continually re-injure your back."

"The drinking and depression was a dangerous medicine you used to save your marriage," the resident explained. "Since you each have genetic susceptibility to one of these disorders, you managed to save your marriage, yet acquire additional diseases. We'll have to treat both of them very aggressively."

With this pronouncement, the initial elation from reuniting gave way to a greater sense of urgency and seriousness. The resident then stressed the life-threatening risks of depression and alcoholism, reciting a litany of sordid case histories that he had treated unsuccessfully. To boost their knowledge regarding the disease processes involved in depression and alcoholism, the resident ordered a "homework" assignment. Mr. Kilroy was instructed to prepare a report from the library about alcoholism, while Mrs. Kilroy was to prepare a similar report about serious depression. An effect of the homework was an increased commitment by each of the spouses to help the other "survive their disease."

Both spouses responded remarkably well to brief problem-focused marital therapy. They began attending 12-Step self-help groups, where they gained more "insight" regarding their "diseases." Mr. Kilroy began to attribute much of his depression to "being a codependent," and also being an adult child of an alcoholic father. He remained on medications for the first time in his life, since "The Program (ACOA) tells you not to play doctor with yourself." Mrs. Kilroy took readily to AA, although stated that "I'm not a typical alcoholic."

Marital therapy was terminated after 12 sessions, with four more booster sessions during the following year. Eight months later, Mr. Kilroy's MAO inhibitor was discontinued. The family has remained "hospital-less" for seven years.

CRISIS INTERVENTION WITH TREATMENT RESISTANT FAMILIES

An irony of family therapy is that while therapists spend substantial time managing crises, many family therapists prefer to make initial contact during a crisis with only one family member. Work with families such as the Kilroys has convinced us that family intervention is absolutely necessary to break the cycle of crisis-proneness and subsequent treatment refusal or failure.

Family intervention during the first crisis session is important for any family suspected of being either treatment resistant or crisis-prone. This is true for a number of reasons. As noted above, individuals in crisis are typically unreliable historians and may not accurately reflect their clinical conditions. Often, individuals who are upset do not process information adequately and may confuse essential details. People in crisis may also be prone to confabulate. For example, the anorexic claims he or she is eating, the schizophrenic claims to be taking medication as prescribed, or the substance abuser claims to be attending self-help meetings and staying straight. Often, individuals are not even aware of their distortions of their present behaviors. Multiple perspectives are extremely useful in formulating a formal psychiatric diagnosis as well as in developing a plan to manage the symptoms.

Because of the fact that families often confuse perceptual and instrumental crises, the degree of instrumentality of a given crisis cannot be adequately assessed without interviewing several family members. It is critically important the therapist interview as many persons in the family as feasible to obtain as accurate a history as possible.

In hospitals and emergency clinics that do not involve families, confusion regarding the degree of instrumentality of the crisis at hand can be common. For example, we are aware of a case where a veteran with Post-Traumatic Stress Disorder was hospitalized for a recurrence of severe flashbacks of a burning village. The veteran claimed that his own apartment had been on fire and that he had to return to his neighborhood to help his family. This was seen as evidence of a reactive psychosis in response to flashbacks and he was treated with a heavy regimen of phenothiazines. Three days later, when the veteran's family was finally interviewed, they revealed the precipitant of this deterioration was an actual fire in the family's apartment that left them homeless.

Another problem with individually oriented crisis intervention–especially of the resistant family–is that it sets an unhealthy precedent. It reinforces family mythology–all too common–that an outside agent will fix the aberrant individual with minimal family effort. Therapy becomes like karate or ballet lessons–merely an activity for the IP while the rest of the family goes about their routine affairs. The family is encouraged to continue patterns of behaviors with the added safety valve of threatening the IP with "a visit to that shrink" if he or she is disobedient or behaves inappropriately. In this vein therapy is seen as punitive social control.

More importantly, individual intervention also makes little theoretical sense for the practicing family therapist. In general, family therapists typically believe the family system either causes or helps maintain the symptom precipitating a crisis. A variety of theories converge on this shared belief. For example, according to strategic theory a depressed adolescent may exhibit symptoms to deflect attention from parental marital discord. A structural account might postulate this depression to be a function of hierarchical disturbance. A systemic behavioral analysis would likely accentuate reinforcing factors in the family's management of the depressed adolescent, such as secondary gains associated with absence from school or the fact his parents allow him to spend weekends alone with his girlfriend "to cheer him up." An assessment of the IP alone, or even the IP followed by the family, rarely results in provision of this type of crucial information. Diagnostic formulations following an initial individual interview are often less important than observation of and understanding the family dynamics in operation (Keeney, 1982). This is especially important in the case of clients who repeatedly present in crisis and then fail to comply with treatment.

Perhaps the most significant reason we endorse family therapy for the resistant family is that individually oriented approaches do not seem effective. For example, the usual individual treatment plan for chronic crisis clients who subsequently resist treatment involves establishing a behavioral contract regarding use of emergency services. The delicate goal of the behavioral contract lies in rewarding the desired behavior of not using emergency services, while simultaneously allowing the client access to such services in a "genuine" emergency. Generally, the reward for desired behavior involves additional staff time, or the right to talk with a particularly favored therapist on a regular basis. The reward value to the client or client family for this class of reinforcers is probably highly inconsistent. Not surprisingly, these types of behavioral contracts are often ineffective.

Some practitioners believe that a successful solution lies in restriction of service utilization. For example, families with a history of entry termination may have their clinical records placed in a special file indicating they are to receive only brief intervention and minimal services. Often, the individual client or family may be seen for an emergency evaluation only after he or she contacts a regular therapist. The therapist must first "authorize" that the client or family can be evaluated. Occasionally these procedures are effective. However, their behavioral nature requires absolute adherence by the entire treatment community to ensure consistency. Often, the family simply finds another agency that will reward them. The case study below highlights this point.

Case Study 4.2. Stan Dong

Stan Dong, a 44-year-old Asian-American man diagnosed as having panic attacks, was placed on restricted access to a community mental health center's after-hours service. Prior to this restriction, he had presented in crisis, either by telephone or in person, an average of five times a month. Medication, including antidepressants and benzodiazepines, proved ineffective in controlling these panic episodes.

Since his therapist believed that family upheavals precipitated his panic attacks, a further restriction placed on Stan was that his wife accompany him to each emergency session. Stan especially disliked this provision and made numerous excuses for why his family shouldn't be involved "in my own little problem." Angry that "No one helps me like I need here," Stan ceased calling in crisis and eventually terminated from therapy completely.

However, once restricted from the mental health center, Stan found other places to meet his needs for crisis intervention. These included two hospitals, another county's crisis intervention services, and a religious-oriented private mental health center where, as Stan astutely noted, "They feel guilty telling me to go away." Each one of these agencies agreed to see him alone and without his wife being present. Eventually he resumed therapy at this latter facility, where the therapist hypothesized that Stan's panic attacks were related to his relations at home. The cycle of restriction of services, termination, and establishment of services elsewhere was repeated again by Stan.

THE GOAL OF CRISIS INTERVENTION WITH RESISTANT FAMILIES

A number of authors have suggested helpful theoretical frameworks for crisis family work. For example, Oster and Caro's (1990) useful model provides three stages of a family crisis interview. These include: (1) understanding the family crisis from the family's perspective; (2) expanding the frame of conceptualization of the crisis; and (3) exploring the pathways of safety and empowering the parents to provide them.

Similarly, Brendler, Silver, Haber, and Sargent (1989), commenting on explosive families, suggest that the goal of the crisis session with a family is both acceptance of the family and disorienting a family from its pathological processes. These are excellent guidelines that we will later build on, but they may not be sufficiently universal. For example, they are irrelevant to the family whose member has just received an AIDS diagnosis or just learned that a child has been sexually molested.

Most of the clinical guidelines for crisis intervention are confusing because they do not make a distinction between crises that evoke a need for support, and crises that warrant a degree of more forceful intervention regarding family processes. Consequently, some authors suggest that the first crisis interview should be used to destabilize the family's hierarchy, or to encourage open expressions of hostility to enable the therapist to obtain a true picture of the family's functioning. The novice or even experienced therapist who attempts these maneuvers with a family that includes a first break schizophrenic youth or an elderly parent who has demonstrated an insidious Alzheimer's-related memory impairment or decline in reasoning capacity may inadvertently commit a serious therapeutic error.

As useful as these other models of crisis intervention are, we advocate a slightly different framework for intervening with resistant systems. The next few chapters will highlight our specific intervention sequences. Here, our discussion is limited to the major guidelines that shape our strategy with difficult families. Our most important goal in intervening with potentially resistant families, especially during crises, is to do no harm. We must recognize that the initial interview may be our sole opportunity to make contact with the resistant system. Therefore, we wish to avoid interventions designed to destabilize or otherwise increase the stress on the family system. Our rationale is that such techniques may continue to work long after the family has abruptly and prematurely terminated treatment.

Our second goal is to actively defuse excessive family tensions and stresses. Because of opponent processes, excessive family tension generates excessive family resistance. It also interferes with problem solving and the ability of family members to adequately assess the severity of their current obstacles. Tension also interferes with communication and fosters an even greater degree of crisis-proneness. While there are some exceptions to this general rule, we will devote substantial energy to reducing family tension and stress prior to other steps with the resistant family.

Our third goal is to empower the family to solve its own problems as much as possible. This may seem to conflict with the needs of keeping the treatment resistant family in therapy. Actually, it does not. By teaching families that they can solve their own problems, family tension is reduced and they will function more appropriately. Moreover, the energy exerted in coping with day-to-day dysfunctional behaviors can be redirected toward addressing more permanent and enduring difficulties. Resistant families (as well as crisis-prone and high risk systems) will rarely make serious progress in therapy as long as they remain dominated by perceptual difficulties. Empowering families to solve their own problems reduces the capacity of perceptual stresses to provoke crises.

Additional specific goals were discussed in Chapter Three. These include encouraging mutual problem solving and reiterating the seriousness of the problem at hand. They also include reducing dysfunctional coping, a technique to be discussed below.

DYSFUNCTIONAL COPING
AND TREATMENT RESISTANCE

In Chapter Three we discussed the finding that resistant families possess more homeostatic mechanisms than crisis-prone families and more functional families. These former families also generally perceive their social, familial, and community supports as more adequate, and hence resist extraneous interventions designed to boost their functioning following turbulent periods. This is one reason the enthusiasm for professional intervention quickly fades with these families and they become treatment resistant.

In recent years research has focused on the process of the family coping with stress and change as a major homeostatic device. Families attempt a variety of coping mechanisms to meet major adaptive tasks. However, systems differ in their ability to pursue the goal of adaptation, based upon their level of functionality. Along these lines, McCubbin and Figley (1983) distinguish between functional and dysfunctional styles of coping. These are summarized in Table 4.1.

Our research suggests that resistant families demonstrate higher numbers of dysfunctional coping mechanisms (McCown & Johnson, 1992c). We found a positive correlation ($r = .39$) between an aggregate measure of treatment resistance and the number of dysfunctional coping mechanisms that a family employs. Indeed, clinical experience suggests that it is rare to find a resistant family that does not employ three or four of these dysfunctional stress-reducing styles. The existence of an abundance of dysfunctional coping mechanisms, combined with the family's relative satisfaction with existing homeostatic supports, tends to readily restore the family to previous equilibrium following a crisis. Figure 4.1 illustrates the manner in which these mechanisms serve to rapidly return a resistant family to its previous level of functioning following a period of change.

In contrast, the crisis-prone family (and to a lesser extent the high risk family) has fewer coping mechanisms and less satisfaction with existing supports. Once a crisis or extreme stressor impacts on the system, there is much less homeostatic "pull" toward previous levels of functioning. This is illustrated in Figure 4.2.

The problem with dysfunctional coping is not that it fails to ameliorate a crisis. It works quite well. However, it works only temporarily. Dysfunctional coping mechanisms foster their own set of problems which frequently precipitate even greater coping problems and eventually crises. To borrow the sociologist Robert Merton's (1968) phrase, dysfunctional coping is *latently* dysfunctional because it works for only a brief period of time before it gives way to something worse. Improper coping maximizes the likelihood that the family system will erupt with additional and greater symptomatology at a later date. This is one reason, we believe, that crisis-proneness and treatment resistance often occur together in families.

In our experience, the therapist of resistant and high risk families cannot prevent the dysfunctional family from employing some or all of their preferred dysfunctional coping mechanisms during a crisis situation. The therapist can, however, challenge the family to use one or more of these adaptive techniques, coaching them during the process and inevitable period of doubt. The successes the family encounters using new methods of dealing with stressors and avoiding former, latently dysfunctional methods can be highlighted–indeed celebrated–by the therapist. When the family has returned to homeostasis other techniques can be taught, modeled, and applied. Ultimately, the family will learn to prevent future crises by maintaining more effective mechanisms of coping.

TABLE 4.1. Functional and Dysfunctional Family Coping

1. *Identification of the Stressor.* Functional families are able to identify and accept what is stressing their social system. Dysfunctional families allow the stressor to remain unclear or, perhaps worse, deny its importance.
2. *Locus of the Problem.* Functional families are able to view the problem as "ours," as a "family problem." Dysfunctional families are more likely to see a problem as outside their onus of responsibility. Dysfunctional families frequently make community agencies or other people responsible for their family's problems.
3. *Approach to the Problem.* Functional families remain solution-oriented and spend collective energy trying to tackle the source of their stressors. Dysfunctional families prefer to spend time, especially in therapy, blaming each other or external agents.
4. *Tolerance of Others.* Functional families are tolerant of others, especially those outside of the family. Dysfunctional families tend to be less tolerant of others, especially of external agencies.
5. *Commitment to and Affection for Family Members.* Functional families are committed to family affection and express it directly and openly. In contrast, dysfunctional families have unclear commitment to other family members and are indirect (or worse) in their expression of affection.
6. *Communication Utilization.* Families who cope functionally are able to communicate with each other effectively and better than families who cope dysfunctionally.
7. *Family Cohesion.* This variable is higher in families who are able to cope functionally. Dysfunctional families may attempt to try to cope by scapegoating or "splitting" the IP from the rest of the family unit. Frequently, they are quick to claim that the family unit is functioning well except for the particular IP.
8. *Family Roles.* McCubbin and Figley state that family roles are flexible and shifting in families that can cope functionally. Rigid and inflexible roles characterize the dysfunctionally coping family.
9. *Resource Utilization.* McCubbin and Figley state that the family that copes functionally is able to utilize its potential resources, or is not afraid to ask for help. The dysfunctionally coping family is unable to do so.
10. *Violence.* Intra and interfamilial violence is disproportionately present in the family that copes dysfunctionally.

11. *Non-Prescription Drugs and Alcohol.* Dysfunctional coping is characterized by the use of nonprescription drugs and habitual excessive episodic alcohol abuse.

After McCubbin and Figley (1983).

MODELS OF FAMILY CRISIS INTERVENTION

During the past several years a variety of models have arisen suggesting steps for family-oriented crisis intervention. For example, Pittman (1987), a pioneer in this field, proposes a seven stage model for treating families in crisis.

Perlmutter and Jones (1986) provide a different sequence, probably more applicable to medical personnel functioning in an emergency room.

Everstine and Everstine (1983) are strategic family therapists

FIGURE 4.1. Resistant Families and Excessive Homeostasis

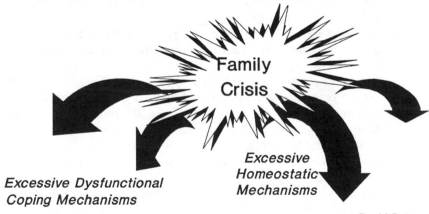

Family Crisis

Excessive Dysfunctional Coping Mechanisms

Excessive Homeostatic Mechanisms

Rapid Return To Pre Crisis State

Previous Level of Family Functioning

FIGURE 4.2. High Risk Families and Homeostasis

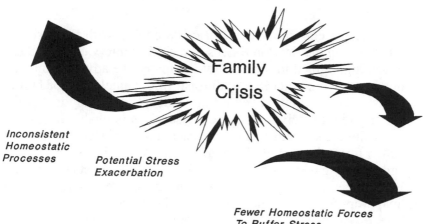

Previous Level of Family Functioning

associated with the MRI who specialize in family emergency intervention. They postulate yet another sequence of steps for family crisis intervention, which we have relied on heavily as well.

Our present method of treatment borrows extensively from each of these models. However, in addition, it is somewhat more tailored for treating families that are likely to be treatment resistant.

Our method is not necessarily mutually exclusive with other conceptualizations and can be juxtaposed with other evaluative and intervention schemas as is appropriate. We differ only in that our emphasis is simultaneously on (1) interventions that can be performed when the family may not return for subsequent treatment and (2) interventions maximizing the likelihood the treatment resistant family will return for additional therapy. It is relatively easy to construct interventions that are appropriate for one of these two goals; however, the real trick is to work at both goals simultaneously. It is with this in mind that our method is perhaps most useful.

CRISIS INTERVENTION
AND CONSULTATION ROLES

How do we enhance successful crisis coping with the resistant family? During the first three steps of the crisis interview with these families, highlighted in the next two chapters, we advocate that the family crisis worker act in a traditional role, namely that of family therapist. The assumption behind the concept of therapy is that the client or patient receiving therapeutic services is unable to resolve distress alone and needs therapy to reach a normal state. In its most common form, the notion of therapy invokes parallels with medical disorders. The patient or family is sick and the therapist acts to cure, or in most cases, to rehabilitate, weakening the family's dependence on inappropriate coping mechanisms in the process.

This quasi-medical model is appropriate for the early stages of family-oriented crisis intervention. The disequilibrium that systems in crisis experience is tantamount to an illness. Crises, like diseases, involve changes that induce abrupt disruption in homeostasis and a deterioration in functioning. The family in crisis may indeed have much in common with a severely ill medical patient. The family as a unit may be unable to reason adequately or, initially, problem solve. The family's capacity to make changes may be limited, and even the ability to accurately report history and presenting problem may be suspect. Left to itself, the family may meet its needs with behaviors that ultimately exacerbate its dysfunction.

Once the family regroups to a level of workable stability, however, we have found it most useful to shift therapeutic gears. The crisis intervention therapist changes roles and becomes a *systems consultant*. The notion of systems consultation to families is one of the most popular developments in family therapy during the last decade. The consultant has an entirely different task than the crisis therapist. He or she functions as an expert in helping the family negotiate the obtainment of their own goals. The consultant no longer thinks of the family as a system in crisis, but instead as a system needing advice and assistance in helping it reach a specific end.

Landau-Stanton (1990) notes the theoretical assumptions involved in the consultation approach with families. The therapist presumes the therapy will be brief, and rapidly engages and then disengages from the system. He or she capitalizes on the family's strengths, rather than their weaknesses. As much as possible, he or she employs the family's natural internal and community supports to allow the family to heal on its own.

Why do we shift roles like this? There are three reasons. The first is pragmatic. Families that are taught to solve their own problems acquire a valuable skill for future use, particularly when the family may not return for treatment. To effectively meet the adaptive tasks a family crisis presents, it may be necessary to intervene aggressively with the family upon the initial contact. The clinician must remember that in many clinical contacts, the client or client family may not return for additional treatment, at least until there is another crisis in the family system. Therefore, there is a substantial chance that the clinician will have only one session to work with the family. Every intervention that the therapist performs should be mindful of this potential limitation. We cannot assume that the family with a history of treatment resistance will return and complete treatment. Therefore, we wish to provide them the experience of generating their own solutions to problems, as much as possible, so they may employ this skill at other times independent of therapeutic presence.

A second reason is more theoretical but just as important. Families are crisis-prone, treatment resistant, or high risk in part because they have an exaggerated response to stressors. They believe that stressors are outside of their control. Often, this is caused or reiterated by their history of psychological trauma or other factors that have caused a sense of powerlessness or learned helplessness. By providing the family with an experience of problem-solving and subsequent family-oriented crisis management, the family is empowered to solve their own crises. Through this mechanism, the controllability and predictability of the family stress is enhanced with consequent decrease in perniciousness of the stress.

A third reason pertains to the practitioners own mental health and well-being. As we indicated in Chapter One, chronic crisis clients and families typically evoke tremendous emotional response from treatment practitioners. Writers such as Barker (1990) emphasize the need for emotional distancing with these patients, implying that the emergency worker should avoid assuming responsibility for failures with this client group. This is especially true for workers attempting to intervene with high risk systems involved in a cycle of crisis and treatment refusal. Crisis workers and family therapists usually hail from a tradition that stresses accountability for therapeutic outcome. For example, authors such as Haley (1976) suggest that therapy failures are usually the responsibility of the therapist and/or supervisor. Although this model may be applicable to prolonged family intervention, it is less applicable to the worker attempting to intervene with resistant systems.

THE STAGES OF THERAPEUTIC/CONSULTATIONAL INTERVENTION

During the initial stages of the crisis session, the worker assumes a traditional therapist role. He or she maneuvers the family to defuse the crisis and to gather necessary information for accurate formulation of the family's problem and generate potential solutions. Then, the worker begins a shift in emphasis. He or she encourages the family to generate their own solutions to their problems and serves as an advisor to assist the family in understanding the reasonableness of their solutions. Dysfunctional coping styles are gently challenged during this period; the crisis worker is acting partly as a therapist and partly as a consultant. Finally, the worker, now acting entirely in a consultant role, attempts to empower the family to carry out their plan and to enhance their ability to solve their own problems in the future.

We have found it useful to work from the following acronym: *ADEPT*, representing the therapist's attempts to (1) *Assemble* the family system together during a crisis (2) *Defuse* the crisis (3) *Evaluate* the family and their problem (4) *Problem-Solve* with the family and finally (5) *Translate* the family's problem solving experience into positive empowerment to solve future problems. As the process continues, the crisis worker acts less as a physician and more of a coach and advisor. Interventions become less frequent and less directive. Communication becomes focused more on facts and rational discourse than on emotion. The "here and now" important during the early stages of the crisis session becomes less important than future plans. Feelings are deemphasized and behaviors are stressed.

CONCLUSION:
SUMMARIZING A NEW STRATEGY
TO UNDERCUT RESISTANCE

To summarize the past two chapters, we argue that families are resistant in part because they have excessive homeostatic mechanisms, usually dysfunctional in nature. These mechanisms encourage the system to disregard the severity of its difficulties and avoid the arduous process of transformation. The clinician intervening with resistant families must work very quickly to establish a "foothold" before the homeostatic processes make these families less amenable to change. One technique useful for doing this is to reduce the aggregate amount of stress that the system is experiencing. Another technique is to gently challenge the usefulness of the coping mechanism for the family. Each of these methods has the goal of circumventing resistance before it arises.

In the next three chapters we will outline a method for engaging resistant families that models itself after many of the methods of crisis intervention. Most of our strategies are similar to those found in traditional family crisis intervention. We want to work quickly, comprehensively, and "ecologically" allowing the family to do as much work on its own as it can.

The reader may have noted a crucial difference between the theory of crisis intervention presented by other practitioners and our goals with resistant families. In traditional crisis intervention, the goal is to work quickly to restore a system to homeostasis. The methods include an emphasis on enhancing family coping and supplementing homeostatic mechanisms with additional interventions that can stabilize the oscillating system. Time is considered crucial, inasmuch as interventions must rapidly return the family to previous levels of functioning before a new and potentially more dysfunctional level of self-organization arises.

In our approach with potentially resistant families we intervene quickly, but for the opposite reason. We are working against excessive homeostatic mechanisms in the resistant system. In other words, we work rapidly *before* the system can be restored to its previous dysfunctional position. We have only a very brief window where we can intervene effectively before the system's overwhelming and conservative forces make more permanent changes unlikely. We therefore negotiate to provide a gentle instability, primarily through weakening the dysfunctional coping styles that impede change.

If we are fortunate, the family will be sufficiently challenged to remain in treatment. If we are extremely fortunate, a new level of self-organization will arise and the family will function in a much better manner, even with minimal intervention. Sometimes–in fact, all too often–our interventions will have been of no apparent value. However, even in this least optimal outcome, we will have provided the family with a potentially positive experience solving its own problems, with minimal reliance on its dysfunctional patterns of crisis response. In any case, we will have done no harm.

Chapter Five

Assembling the Family During Crisis: The First Session

As indicated in Chapter Four, there are several excellent references regarding crisis intervention and family therapy. This book is not intended to duplicate these previous works. Instead, we are primarily concerned with illustrating techniques with specific utility for the resistant system. Many of the most effective techniques the clinician can employ are implemented within the first few minutes of the first session. In fact, the most severe mistakes clinicians make regarding treatment of resistant family systems often occur within the first five minutes of intervention.

The purpose of this chapter is to assist the clinician in avoiding these mistakes. Success or failure with the family is often determined by the manner in which the therapist initially assembles the person or persons who will receive treatment. Proper assembling of the important components of the family system is the first step in helping the dysfunctional family break its cycle of treatment termination. This chapter presents a number of pragmatic concerns regarding this initial step.

FAMILY CRISIS INTERVENTION: WHO SHOULD BE SEEN?

Anytime that *anyone* in the family system is being advised or seen regarding a psychiatric or psychological crisis, the therapist is providing family crisis intervention. Family intervention can be as brief as a single telephone call to a parent, or, in some cases, may extend to many sessions, months, or even years. Family crisis intervention is not restricted only to crisis workers, or even family therapists. The long-term, individually-oriented therapist who responds to a midnight call from an IP's mother is performing family-oriented crisis therapy. Crises inherently involve family members. It is impossible to exclude them, even if one wished to do so. In performing crisis intervention, the question is not "Should I work with the family?" but instead, "Which family members should I work with?"

Before assembling the family for the first session, the family-oriented crisis therapist is confronted with an immediate problem: of all of the available family members, who should participate in the crisis intervention session? The manner in which this question is answered will frequently determine the entire course of crisis resolution and subsequent treatment cooperation.

The first guideline is that as many family members possible should be seen as soon as possible. Without being argumentative, invite everyone who is in the nuclear family to participate in treatment. Notice that we have said "invite," and not "cajole," "force," or "ensnare." It is unusually helpful to minimize the ground rules for family involvement (or as Carl Whitaker might say, the battle for who decides the family involvement) during the initial crisis session. However, moderate firmness in asking for participation is recommended. If other relatives or significant others are intensely involved in the family system, they should be asked to attend the session. Involvement of the entire family sets the stage for the idea a problem is familial, rather than individual. Hence, efforts from the least important or powerful member to the most important and powerful are necessary to overcome the difficulty.

The therapist need not interview each family member if it is inappropriate or unhelpful to do so. Usually, however, every family member should be provided the opportunity to contribute during the first session. These "insignificant others" are most often helpful because their perceptions of the crisis are so different from those of the rest of the family. This is illustrated in the high risk family below.

Family Study 5.1. The Sweeneys

John Sweeney is a 43-year-old chronic schizophrenic who lives with his brother Ted, 39, Ted's wife Joan, 37, and their two children, Ted, Jr. 11, and Adrianne, 7. John apparently had discontinued his medication for the two previous months and deceived the family regarding his present dosage. He was assessed by a social worker at a local mental health clinic who suggested prescreening for involuntary hospitalization due to "exacerbation of hallucinations and violent delusions."

Because she had previously successfully employed family interventions, the social worker decided to ask the other family members about John and his level of functioning. Frankly, she expected this to be merely an academic exercise, since the case was "open and shut." John was well known to her and the clinic. He periodically discontinued his own medications, about once a year or so and most often in the summer. He usually complained that the "pills don't let me sweat right," and since it was July, John's appearance was quite predictable.

Regardless, the social worker talked with each person in the family. She learned little until it was Adrianne's turn to speak. The little girl stated with childhood candidness that "Mommy and me want Uncle John to go back to the hospital so we can go to New York. I love New York and Mommy does, too. Every summer he gets sick so we can go on vacation."

Future therapeutic work with the Sweeneys stressed the need for the family to experience a respite from John's care. It was arranged that John would spend time in the summer with other family members, allowing the Sweeneys to go on vacation.

Excessive pressure regarding attendance at the initial interview can damage needed rapport with resistant families; hence, the wise therapist relents when clinically appropriate. However, the observation of who does not attend despite being asked to do so furnishes important diagnostic information regarding family coalitions or struggles for power that otherwise may not be apparent.

An exception to this "Do not pressure" routine should be made for the father or the male figure in the family system. It is all too easy to get locked into a pattern where the male figure is not involved in family therapy interactions. As the study by Martin (1977) indicates, brief family therapy is much more efficacious if it includes the father. Hence, every effort should be made to persuade the father figure in the family system to participate in the crisis session.

A second exception regards the necessity of seeing the person who initiated the crisis intervention contact. Often–in fact, usually, with the resistant family–this person is not the IP. Oster and Caro (1990) argue that the individual making the initial call should be recognized by the crisis worker as the "designated family spokesperson." This person has an unknown, but apparently important, role in the family and should be included in all family sessions whenever possible. We have found this principle to be extremely important in treating resistant families–especially the high risk family. Ignoring the designated spokesperson portends premature therapy termination.

On the other hand, tendencies on the part of the designated spokesperson to dominate the crisis session must be avoided. Often, designated spokespersons seek to use the session to emotionally "ventilate" or to present a list of alleged infractions by the IP against family rules. Therapy that encourages emotional ventilation without equal emphasis on responsibility and problem solving is usually counterproductive (Stuart, 1980). We will comment more about this in the next chapter.

Novice family therapists often assume that crisis-prone or treatment resistant family members will be reluctant to participate in the initial assembly. Actually, individuals from these systems are frequently *more likely* to participate in the early stages of therapy. Much of the "teeth pulling" necessary to get family members into the therapist's office is not necessary, presumably because the system is spurred into temporary cooperation by the crisis at hand. A polite, but authoritative telephone call is usually all that is necessary to encourage family attendance during acute stages of a family crisis, or during the first therapy interview.

Often, the first contact a resistant family has with mental health agencies is through crisis lines or other telephone counseling services. These programs can be highly effective in providing initial crisis intervention (Hornblow, 1986), given they are properly staffed and implemented. They can also be a conduit for invitation of the entire family system into treatment. We find that resistant families are more likely to come in for subsequent treatment if the telephone crisis worker they have interacted with previously is the worker assigned to them as a regular therapist. When this is impractical or impossible, we have found it helpful if the previous crisis worker provides some contact with the family during the first few treatment sessions. It is also conducive to treatment if the worker telephones the family before the first session with their new therapist and reminds them of their appointment. A call or two after each session is also usually appropriate.

WHO SHOULD SEE RESISTANT FAMILIES?

Obviously, before the family is assembled, a decision needs to be made regarding who will see them. This question actually involves two separate problems: which particular staff persons should see the family and what level of practitioner is appropriate for intervention.

The first question is easiest to answer and hardest to implement. No one should see resistant families unless they believe such families have the capacity to change. Families respond to the negative expectancies of therapists. A therapist who is skeptical about the possibility of a family changing—even if he or she has seen the family twenty times previously in an emergency—should not work with the family. Similarly, if previous unpleasant experiences with a particular family cause hard feelings or "burn out," the therapist should acknowledge this and, if at all possible, avoid intervening with that family.

The question regarding the optimal type of mental health professional for service provision is a complex issue rife with political overtones. Regarding education level, for example, an archival study of 68 high risk family cases from our data base yielded no significant correlation (.06) between the degree of practitioner education and the likelihood the crisis family would return for treatment. In fact, one of the best family crisis workers we know has a General Equivalency Diploma! The issue of psychiatric coverage for crisis-prone and resistant families will be discussed below.

The minimal education requirements for family-oriented workers should emphasize general knowledge rather than formal degrees. It is essential that family crisis specialists possess extensive familiarity with family therapy theory, practice, and crisis intervention theory. Excellent psychodiagnostic skills are also compulsory. All new workers should be extensively supervised, regardless of their academic or clinical credentials. Preferably, this supervision should include team intervention for the first few months.

Although certain crisis workers seem particularly successful at securing cooperation with difficult families, characteristics of these workers remain ill-defined. In all likelihood, characteristics such as empathy, friendliness, persuasiveness, and limit-setting all contribute to the differential effectiveness of these individuals. Obviously, people working with resistant families also need to possess a tremendous capacity to endure the uncontrollable stress usually associated with interviewing, evaluating, and problem solving with a multi-dysfunctional system.

It is important for the worker to realize that his or her skills rapidly grow rusty without frequent use. Unless the family crisis therapist deals with two or three crises a week, he or she will experience some degree of "atrophy of skills." Past experience and academic knowledge of intervention techniques are necessary, but not sufficient, for optimal intervention with high risk families. Crisis intervention with resistant families is similar to surgery, in that the best practitioners are those who perform the task most often.

Perhaps the single most important characteristic of a therapist lies in the capacity to treat dysfunctional and difficult families with dignity. Dignity is one of the harder aspects to inculcate into the treatment regimen. Often the frustrated or harried crisis worker or therapist will inadvertently hurry or slight the family in seemingly innocuous ways. Resistant families are frequently hypersensitive to perceived discourtesies and will readily use them as an excuse to discontinue or avoid treatment.

Prior to seeing a crisis-prone and resistant family, the nonphysician therapist needs to consider the extent of medical backup that might be necessary. Many psychiatrists who work with families that we would consider high risk find it inconceivable that family therapists perform their tasks in the absence of adequate medical backup. Crisis therapists who work under conditions of insufficient medical resources would probably agree, but are nonetheless mandated to do their jobs (Barker, 1990). In an ideal world, therapists would enjoy ready access to physicians and other medical personnel who would respect their expertise, yet be available to provide immediate consultation and intervention regarding medication and other relevant areas. In turn, therapists would be aware of the beneficial aspects of medication in many patients' lives, and would feel comfortable allowing their pharmacologically trained colleagues to perform their multidisciplinary team effort. This ideal is rarely the case today.

Nonmedical therapists functioning outside of a hospital setting may be mistrusted by physicians. The distrust is often mutual, as these workers may view physicians as prone to overmedicating and substituting pills for therapeutic patience and acumen. Both sides may view the other as insensitive to the patients' real needs. Resistant families readily exploit this distrust (Barker, 1990). Based upon the advice of a particular physician that medication may solve their problem, they may balk at the notion of therapy. Or, they may discontinue medications based upon statements or opinions verbalized by the nonmedical professional.

Fortunately, the past decade has seen a growing sentiment that different professionals can offer unique contributions to the care of families in crises. For example, the anti-medication zealousness of some family therapists of the 1970s and early 1980s has been tempered by the realization that many psychiatric disorders require medical treatment (Oster & Caro, 1990). Conversely, physicians are gaining an understanding of the role of systemic factors in precipitating and encouraging both medical and psychiatric crises (Perlmutter & Jones, 1986). Continued progress and mutual understanding may thus promote future greater gain for the client.

Many family therapists routinely work without adequate medical coverage. Some work exceptionally well, even brilliantly. In our experience with hospital deferral programs, we developed the capability to manage a variety of psychiatric crises without medication, at least temporarily (Levy & McCown, 1983). These capabilities included treating violent and homicidal clients, acutely suicidal individuals, decompensating schizophrenics, and even manic depressives. Many patients that otherwise would have been heavily medicated were treated with verbal therapies in the context of the family crisis. As indicated in Chapter Four, the family can be encouraged to successfully manage some disorders at home, rather than in the hospital.

Despite some of these successes, we cannot recommend that crisis workers be required to perform such interventions on a routine basis. In our experience, medication issues are important in approximately 15 percent of crises involving resistant families. Hence, adequate medical, and preferably psychiatric, coverage is necessary.

Non-physician crisis workers generally encounter two major issues when discussing family treatment problems with physicians. The first involves the general perceived competency of nonmedical health care professionals. Usually time and a working alliance can ameliorate this problem. A second problem is more difficult to solve. Physicians often have little training in the understanding of the role of systemic factors in promoting psychiatric crises. Older, analytically trained psychiatrists may be particularly antagonized by the therapist's insistence upon treating the family, rather than the individual patient. Careful description of the populations that are being served and the interventions offered will help prevent professional conflict. Of course, modesty, as opposed to hubris, is no doubt important.

Some of the best routinely available medical coverage for crisis services is connected with the recent upsurge of private crisis phone lines established by for-profit psychiatric hospitals. When the motive for such services is one of genuine altruism and a desire for community services, these facilities have a positive impact upon the community. In our experience, however, some of these crisis lines are little more than high pressure advertisements and conduits for particular inpatient facilities. Crisis workers may even have monthly patient hospitalization quotas to fill. This state of affairs will likely continue until regulating agencies or professional bodies put an end to such practices.

LOCATION OF THE CRISIS SESSION

Another basic question that has to be addressed before the family is assembled is "Where is the best location for evaluating a resistant family system in crisis?" Many crisis workers, especially those who "think systemically," believe that it is necessary to assess and intervene in the family's natural setting, i.e., in the home or community. Others, perhaps wary of the potential danger of such a location, disagree. They may also argue that the family who is unwilling to come to a community agency for intervention is not likely to be compliant with treatment recommendations and further sessions.

During the 1970s and early 1980s the concept of a "Mobile Crisis Team" was popular with mental health professionals. Many crisis agencies, such as the ones the authors were affiliated with during this period, performed assessment and intervention in community settings. Often, the therapist's "office" was the home of the person or system in crisis. Crisis therapists frequently worked in locations that were often new to them. These included transient hotels, establishments catering to drug users, and taverns or other social facilities. An excellent description of the methods of a family-oriented mobile crisis team is available in the work by Everstine and Everstine (1983). Another useful work regarding general family therapy outreach is contained in Clark, Zalis, and Sacco (1982).

There are several advantages of mobile crisis teams (Bengelsdorf & Alden, 1987). One advantage is that they broaden outreach ability for clients who are otherwise too paranoid, hostile, or confused to present for necessary mental health services. A second advantage is that they encourage clients to discuss their problems in a natural setting, where presumably they are less defensive and perhaps more forthcoming. A third advantage is that the systems-oriented crisis worker is able to obtain an *in vivo* snapshot of the clients' home and family life (Clark, Zalis, & Sacco, 1982). The information gained by this type of on-site intervention was often invaluable for future treatment planning.

Unfortunately, there is usually risk associated with on-site interventions. This is especially the case when systems are treatment resistant or individuals harbor animosity or suspicion towards mental health professionals. Furthermore, many mental health agencies have curtailed the budgets of emergency services, mandating that a single crisis worker handle interventions on site. This multiplies the danger to the crisis worker. Problems with insurance reimbursement and professional liability have further restricted the feasibility of community crisis intervention. Finally, the societal upsurge in drug use and violence has complicated on-site intervention for even the most well-equipped and best trained crisis teams.

Because of these and other factors we can no longer advocate home or community assessment and intervention into family crises. Although our clinical impressions indicate these interventions to be often extremely useful for encouraging subsequent treatment compliance of resistant systems, we have seen no reliable data to convince us the benefits offset the risks. However, the worker should be aware that the site where he or she is working functions as a prescreen in determining what types of cases are seen. For example, hospital emergency rooms are much more likely to see patients experiencing substance abuse problems and major psychiatric disorders than community mental health centers, crisis lines, and family counseling services. Hospital emergency rooms are also more likely to see clients with instrumental crises. Finally, clients who present to emergency rooms with perceptual crises in general have a lengthy history of crisis-proneness and treatment noncompliance.

TIMING AND LENGTH OF SESSIONS
AND CRISIS INTERVENTION

When we refer to a *crisis intervention process* we mean the completion of all activities specified by our acronym ADEPT; that is (1) assembling the family (2) defusing the crisis (3) evaluating the family (4) problem solving and finally, (5) translating the problem solving success into future empowerment. Individual crisis sessions, on the other hand, refer to the length of time the worker or therapist is physically administering services to the family, either in person or on the telephone. As we have shown in Chapter One, resistant families often will fail to return for more than two or three sessions. Therefore we attempt to conclude this entire *ADEPT* process in *at most* two or three sessions.

Prior to assembling the family for the initial session the therapist needs to consider the timing and length of his or her potential interventions. Foremost is the necessity to schedule a potentially resistant family quickly. A family suspected of being in crisis should be seen as soon as possible. This point may seem self-evident. However, many client families, even in private clinics, have described placement on waiting lists during crisis periods. This is problematic for several reasons. First is the obvious emergency nature of the family's problem. A family in crisis may behave dangerously and unpredictably. Secondly, a family in crisis is often a motivated family. For maximal efficacy, the therapist must "strike while the iron is hot" before faulty homeostatic patterns arise to institutionalize the dysfunctional behavior. Delays in initial intervention correlate with subsequent treatment resistance. Therefore, the family needs to be seen as soon as possible.

Consideration should also be given to session length, especially for the first session. Sessions that are too long encourage subsequent client "no show" before the problem is resolved. Sessions that are too short encourage the family believe that they have not been treated sincerely and fairly. There are no firm rules regarding optimal session length. We have performed family crisis intervention with resistant systems in individual sessions as brief as twenty minutes and for as long as five hours. More extended time periods are usually indicated for systems that are longer or more complex. Clinical judgment is necessary for each case. Naturally, it is an inappropriate expectation on the part of the therapist to believe that he or she can perform satisfactory crisis resolution with various families if they are scheduled "back-to-back" in fifty-minute time slots. Agencies mandating that emergency workers schedule crisis cases in this manner are doing their clients a disservice.

In general, more experienced therapists can work more quickly with resistant families in crisis than novices. Through practice, clinical judgment becomes sharpened to the point where noncritical or unnecessary interventions during the crisis are eliminated. However, until the individual clinician is comfortable with an accelerated pace, he or she should be afforded as much time as necessary for intervening with resistant families in crisis. The personality of the therapist may also be important in determining how quickly he or she works with families in crisis. More extroverted therapists tend to work faster, while more introverted therapists prefer a slower pace. As long as families do not feel they are being rushed or slighted, there is little correlation between the length of sessions and the likelihood the family will comply with treatment recommendations or subsequent treatment efforts.

HANDLING ANGER OF THE RESISTANT FAMILY

The family therapist intervening with resistant families will routinely encounter varying degrees of anger directed towards him or her. As a rule, this anger is the greatest problem during the first few minutes of the initial session, where all family members are assembled together and expected to behave with civility toward each other and the therapist. Perlmutter and Jones (1986), physicians who specialize in emergency consultation with families in crisis, note that dysfunctional families in crisis often express extreme hostility toward emergency workers. They note it "becomes clear that (some families have) a need to project years of pent-up rage at the staff no matter what is done" (p. 117). They highlight the "inevitable dysphoria of such a scene," ending with the "interviewer feeling trapped, de-skilled and helpless" (p. 116).

However, Perlmutter and Jones are more optimistic that systemic involvement, including as many family members as feasible, can help reduce this anger towards the emergency professional. We agree. In our experience, the more family members involved in initial consultation, the less anger is apt to be displayed by the system toward the therapist. Anger generally is less of a problem in later stages of the first interview, in subsequent interviews, or in later work with the family.

Regardless, however, there will be many instances when resistant families leave dissatisfied and angry regarding the treatment they have received from therapists and their agencies. Therapists and their supervisors need to be mindful of this tendency and to adjust their expectations accordingly. For example, one of the authors was once "reported" to the state governor's office by a high risk alcoholic family who demanded a seventh inpatient treatment (in two years) be provided *at public expense* for an inebriated son. Clinically, this was a completely inappropriate request, as the whole family consistently colluded to sabotage the brief sobriety of their son. Fortunately, there were no public beds available in the state at the time, but the family was not mollified. The author had to review the case with a bureaucrat from the governor's office for five hours, in order to effectively address the complaints of the family.

COMMUNICATION PRINCIPLES
DURING CRISIS INTERVENTION

While the resistant family is being assembled it is often helpful to remember that individuals and systems that are under stress may experience difficulty in communicating. This typically includes problems associated with anger and heightened emotional states, resulting in distorted verbal and nonverbal communications. Along these lines, Everstine and Everstine (1983) discuss communication principles found useful in high stress or dangerous situations. Use of these principles appears to enhance communications with families and reduce the anger felt toward the therapist. They also appear to enhance the probability the high risk family will be treatment compliant and return for subsequent sessions. Ten of these principles are listed in Table 5.1. below. A more thorough discussion of them is available in the book by Everstine and Everstine.

TABLE 5.1. Principles of Communication for Crisis Situations

1. Speak in a language and style congruent with the client family's.
2. Early in the process, get the family to agree with trivial statements. It is important to get the family "used to saying yes."
3. Focus on behavior. Do not presume to understand what other people are feeling unless you ask or they tell you.
4. Avoid exaggerated statements, such as "always," "never," "hardly ever" and "all."
5. Keep communications simple and direct.
6. Be polite and reasonable.
7. Communicate humbly, using phrases such as "I will try" or "I'll do what I can" rather than guaranteeing results.
8. Be realistic.

9. Be empathetic.
10. Be supportive, and use praise cautiously.

After Everstine and Everstine (1983).

Often, stress levels and negative affect cannot easily be reduced to the level where the therapist can intervene in an attempt to enhance the family's coping capacity. In this case, the therapist must maintain either covert or overt ground rules to govern family interaction. Both novice and experienced crisis therapists frequently overlook this important point. The results become chaotic, as four or five family members simultaneously clamor for the floor, or take turns swearing at each other.

To minimize this in an effort to propel the family toward coping, we suggest a minimum number of rules to include the following:

1. Only one individual should be allowed to talk at any time. Interruptions will be politely but firmly stopped.
2. All family members must be respectful to each other. The use of profanity should be discouraged. (This is a rule we did not enforce until recently. The liberal use of profanity in many of our family studies should convince the therapist of the need for this rule.)
3. The therapist should gently insist that discussion be related to present and relevant past behaviors, with no attribution regarding motives.
4. Unless the therapist has strong reason to suspect the family of collusion, all information should be presented in a familial context. (Exceptions regarding child abuse and incest are discussed later.)

It is often helpful for the therapist to articulate that she or he will see each family member privately for no more than a minute or two at the end of each session. This injunctive discourages commonly encountered tendencies toward triangling and splitting. It also discourages excessive ventilating by the long-suffering spouse or child, which we do not believe is appropriate at this point of family treatment.

It is entirely appropriate for families who may violate these rules to be politely told of them in advance. Setting limits on families during emergency situations is one of the most difficult skills to master. Often, a power struggle will emerge between a family member and the limit-setting therapist. A less intrusive manner of circumventing this struggle (rather than abrupt verbal reminders) is to prominently display a copy of the "therapy rules." This strategy is also helpful for working with concrete families, or with troubled adolescents who may want to know where the rules are written down. In highly chaotic families, it may be necessary to briefly outline the rules before the family session begins. Often, a signature of all members of the family on a copy of the rules is beneficial.

Almost invariably, someone in the resistant family will deliberately violate the rules. When this occurs, it is usually helpful if the therapist assumes a "one down" position, and takes responsibility for the fact the family is refusing to abide by the previously stated rules. An example is demonstrated below, subsequent to a disruptive and intense verbal altercation between two parents regarding a suicidal young man.

Family Study 5.2. The Spaldings

Mother (regarding her teenage son): It's worse than that. It really is. I can't tell you in front of the other children, but as soon as we talk together, I mean you and me personal (sic) I could fill that file of yours over there with the things he does.

Therapist (to the mother): Well, as we said, that's against the rules. Remember, we agreed to discuss everything together. That's my fault (to the entire family). I apologize, folks. I really do. I'm afraid I didn't make myself clear about the rules. This is a very hard time for all of us . . . Why don't I post the rules in the center of the table so we all can remember them? That way we'll be working together.

Mother: No, it . . . I mean, well . . . I expect him to follow rules and I guess I should, too. And if it's a rule in writing, it must be a good one, one that helps people.

With the rules posted in this manner, the therapist can enable the person breaking them to realize their infraction. This strategy works best with an adolescent. An inoffensive and often effective way of limiting a child or adolescent's behavior is to have a sibling "flag" the infracted rule. For example, children might be given a buzzer to ring when an adolescent brother uses profanity. The levity of this procedure often builds rapport and encourages the family to monitor its own behavior.

Once the crisis is resolved and (if!) the family enters ongoing therapy, this procedure can be easily adapted and made more interesting by fining family members a nominal sum for rule infraction within the session. This works especially well when a dysfunctional family has been given a set of behavioral rules to follow in and outside of the session. Reinforcement during the session, especially by children, is a powerful technique to promote generalization. Children can be quite vigilant when given a nickel or dime for every infraction they find. Their enthusiasm and playfulness may buffer some of the anger family members may experience about having their behaviors observed and operantly reinforced. Our experience is that this procedure works less well outside of the office, except for discrete behaviors such as smoking or cursing. Dysfunctional families are much less able to use this procedure outside of the office, although their overall generalization of training seems equivalent to more functional groups. Care needs to be taken when using this strategy with parents, to avoid undermining their authority.

PAYMENT OF FEES

Therapists usually are not comfortable discussing fees. This is even more likely when the therapist must intervene with a resistant family. Many resistant families have little income and simply cannot pay much, if anything. In today's economic marketplace, such families receive few services, except perhaps at the local emergency room (Perlmutter & Jones, 1986).

It is essential that the therapist resolve ambivalence regarding fees *prior* to assembling the potentially resistant family. Questions regarding fees should be addressed honestly so that problems are minimized and an unexpected surprise regarding their existence is not used by the family as an excuse to terminate treatment.

One of the most discouraging scenarios is when a family presents in crisis and appears to have the capacity for therapeutic growth. However, upon inquiry regarding mental health insurance they find their coverage does not allow further treatment. Billing and insurance reimbursement are often issues used by high risk families in crises to avoid treatment. Sometimes these are merely excuses, but increasingly, this problem reflects reality and is often insurmountable.

We are aware of the dilemmas the practitioner confronts when free or reduced-fee treatment is provided while business pressures and costs mount. Unfortunately, we have no magic solutions. The decision to evaluate and treat difficult families is not usually made for financial gain, but instead out of compassion and clinical necessity. However, in our experience as private practitioners, we find substantially fewer uncollectible bills from our caseload when we specify *in advance* that families will be seen only for a limited number of sessions. We also estimate the expense associated with such treatment and inform the family of projected cost. One distinct advantage to a consultation and crisis intervention model is that it tends to reduce the probability that a large number of families will accumulate exorbitant bills they can ill afford.

We have found it a useful practice to contract to see the client family for a reduced number of sessions (usually three) regardless of insurance coverage or ability to pay. During this period, we may encourage the client family to seek alternative referrals. Quite often, the family will "discover" that their insurance policy really does allow coverage. Or, they will agree to pay with funds earmarked for other sources. For example, a portion of vacation money may be used for brief therapy. In our experience, resistant and high risk families sometimes make more progress once they are paying out of pocket.

Some practitioners believe that all families should make at least a token payment. In general, the literature has failed to support the notion that payments are related to therapeutic progress. However, such studies are conducted primarily on persons in individual therapy and may not be applicable to families. What *is* clearly helpful in reducing abrupt "no shows" in resistant families is charging the family when they *miss* a session, unless, of course, sufficient notice is given.

HOSPITALIZATION

This chapter closes with a topic that some family therapists may consider unpleasant: hospitalization of the IP. Many family-oriented crisis therapists consider hospitalization a dirty word. The very mention of it, for some people, is an indication that the therapist is unskilled or performed clumsily. Worse, it is seen as a failure of the entire paradigm of family therapy theory! However, hospitalization is a common occurrence with resistant family systems and is sometimes inevitable. The decision whether to hospitalize an IP is usually made following the initial family assembly. This is true in all but the most salient cases where a decision may be made on the basis of police report or testimony of family or neighbors obtained via telephone. In most cases where the emergency therapist is not a physician, a medical doctor will be required to "certify" or otherwise approve of the decision to hospitalize. Often, these persons have little or no recent training in mental health, and especially, in systems-oriented crisis intervention. Sometimes they simply complicate the family system further by undermining the carefully planned strategy of the therapist. Negative experiences with such physicians frequently cause the nonmedical worker to further avoid the possibility of resorting to hospitalization.

Unfortunately, there are no absolute "right or wrongs" regarding the appropriateness of hospitalization. Each case is different. Laws ranging by jurisdiction preclude a "cookbook" approach to the question of when to hospitalize. Many systems, such as overburdened urban hospitals, also have unwritten rules regarding when the clinician should hospitalize an IP. Usually, the decision to hospitalize is ambiguous and comes down to a "judgment call." As limited as clinical judgment may occasionally be, there is frequently little substitute for it.

More experienced family therapists often will avoid the decision to hospitalize until they have assembled and evaluated the family on several occasions. Sometimes this works well with the resistant family, who will suddenly "solve" their problem rather than submit to additional therapy. However, novice crisis therapists often go to inappropriate lengths to avoid hospitalization. Occasionally, these techniques work brilliantly for keeping people out of the hospital.

When there are no beds available, heroic efforts are sometimes mandated, even on a routine basis.

However, we maintain a conservative position with regard to hospitalization and the resistant family. Hospitalization is always mandated when the IP is in imminent danger to self or others. This is the law in most states and countries. It is much better to err on the side of caution here. Competent family therapists must be able to make routine psychiatric diagnostic assessments, assess lethality, and ascertain mental status. They must also be willing to "make the call" when they believe a client is a danger to self and/or others.

Secondly, further evaluation and possible hospitalization should always be considered when there is a new, *sudden* and deleterious change in the IP's affect or thought processes. We have seen too many "systems" cases that had underlying medical etiologies. For example, a systemically oriented physician colleague used family therapy in treatment of the 14-year-old daughter of a woman with chronic lupus. The complaining problem of the IP was a rapid onset depression with vegetative signs. It seemed like a "perfect family case." The young woman was eventually found to have a glioblastoma (brain tumor) and died.

From a systems perspective, hospitalization of the IP in a resistant family presents an opportunity for an invaluable diagnostic family experiment. Once a disruptive patient is removed from the home environment (and if our hypotheses regarding patient symptoms serving some familial function are true) we should see a deterioration in the functioning of another family member or other index of family functioning. On the other hand, if family functioning improves, we have evidence for the hypothesis that the family system's aberrant behavior is a *response* to the individual psychopathology of the IP, rather than a contributor or cause.

Family Study 5.3. Gerald Henley

Gerald Henley is a 55-year-old African-American veteran with a diagnosis of chronic schizophrenia. He has been hospitalized 11 times since he was first diagnosed at age 21.

Despite his disease, Gerald has made a satisfactory adjustment to the community. Until the past two years he has been employed as a security guard. He has remained married for 28 years and has four children, all of whom appear in reasonable mental health. He is a deacon of his church and is active in community and youth groups. He has been conscientious regarding medication and outpatient therapy, although recently both his therapist and his medication physician observe a decrease in his cooperation and overall functioning.

Following consultation with the family, Gerald is hospitalized at the VA hospital psychiatry unit. A therapist assigned to the case consults with the family and asks them to informally monitor their daily stress levels. While Gerald is hospitalized, the family reports progressively less daily anxiety and stress. The therapist consults with the family on a weekly basis. Family functioning is improving in Gerald's absence. Cynthia, his wife, reports feeling extremely guilty about her husband's absence, but also notes that she is happy that her husband is hospitalized and out of the home. The children also report less tension at home.

Gerald is discharged six weeks later with little noticeable improvement. Once he is home, the family reports a decrease in pleasantness and an increase in stress.

Our formulation with Cynthia and Gerald is that the family system is reacting to Gerald's condition, rather than causing it. Subsequent neuropsychological testing indicates that Gerald is in the early stages of an Alzheimer's-type dementia superimposed on the schizophrenia.

Another type of family shows symptom substitution or deterioration following hospitalization of the IP. This is usually characteristic of the high risk family.

Family Study 5.4. John Havermyer and Family

John is a 44-year-old Caucasian veteran who was admitted to a VA hospital following a suicide attempt. During this hospitalization, he tells the attending physician that he attempted suicide because he has been having intercourse with his 13-year-old daughter, Sandy. His wife, Julie, 39, appears to be "in denial" regarding this and has attempted to ignore the very obvious clues regarding her husband's behavior. An older daughter Mary, 20, also lives at home and reports to the attending physician that she too was sexually abused until age 18.

Upon investigation by a family services social worker, both daughters report relief their Dad is in the hospital. The mother is ambivalent. However, the two boys in the family, John Jr., 15, and Jake, 12, have become "unmanageable" during the father's absence. John Jr. was arrested for stealing a car. Jake has attempted on three occasions to beat Sandy, calling her a "tattling whore" and "crazy slut."

Following her father's hospitalization, Mary has shown several instances of extremely bad judgment regarding her personal safety. These include picking up intoxicated hitchhikers, having sex with strangers, and driving around alone in very bad parts of town.

In the case of the Havermeyers, we may hypothesize with a greater degree of certainty that the family's problems are not limited to incest. Nor will they necessarily disappear if the incest ceases or if the perpetrator vanishes. We do not know exactly what the difficulty is; however, through this experience we can see that the father's presence has a stabilizing influence on the family system.

With inpatient treatment programs there is often a rush to immediately begin family work. One reason, obviously, is that limited stays of patients mandate that as much therapy be "crammed" into as few hospital days as possible. A second, less therapeutic reason is that such therapy is usually reimbursable, thus serving as one way to generate revenue. From a family therapist's viewpoint, there may be strong theoretical reasons *not* to treat the resistant family during inpatient hospitalizations. The therapist might be more effective with limited contact with the family, and requesting them to monitor their own functioning during the patient's absence.

Chapter Six

Crisis Defusion and Evaluation

Our first treatment goal with resistant families is to enhance family coping with present stressors. This goal is not unique to our approach. Enhanced family coping is a popular aim for therapists working in a variety of modalities, including longer-term family therapies. Unfortunately, attainment of this goal becomes more challenging when the system is treatment resistant or otherwise noncompliant. Therefore, our task is to find techniques that will work quickly with families, allowing them to enhance their own coping. At the same time such techniques should not lead to an increased dependence of the family on professional help. Interventions that work too well could backfire, leading the family to call a therapist every time they experience a routine stressor.

This chapter discusses the next two steps in our process of fostering adaptive response to family stress. These steps involve the dual task of crisis defusion and subsequent evaluation of the family system. Both are performed quickly, and relatively discretely. Both steps are also essential before the family can begin to enhance its own functional coping styles.

CRISIS DEFUSION (D): MAKING THE CRISIS "WORKABLE"

In order to allow the restorative process, the therapist must often provide initial defusion of the current situation. Defusion simply means letting the hostile energy in the family system dissipate so that the real purpose of the crisis intervention can be found. The goal of defusion is that *enough* of the hostility, anger, hopelessness, rage, and general discouragement that the family possesses can be *temporarily* overcome so that other necessary steps can be implemented to allow a successful resolution of the crisis. This goal must be viewed in the context of the family as a complex system. Too much or premature defusion can encourage subsequent crisis-proneness by destroying the purpose of the crisis for the system. It also can encourage the family to seek unneeded interventions any time it wishes to "ventilate." The art of crisis intervention is in providing just enough defusion to keep the family workable during their crisis.

Defusion involves a number of possible interventions. It may begin on the telephone when the therapist's reassuring voice and manner serves to reduce systemic tensions. Defusion is accentuated when the system realizes that the therapist is competent and caring enough to see them quickly and is genuinely interested in their problems. However, the process of defusion usually will not be successful until the system is interviewed by the therapist and each member of the system has a chance to comment on the crisis at hand.

It is presumed the therapist will have established rapport sufficient to facilitate communications between all members of the crisis family. In extreme cases, or cases with substantial family pathology, it may be impossible to reduce familial stress to the point where family members interact with one another. However, families will almost always speak with a therapist in emergency situations, even if they are at fisticuffs with each other and the rest of the world.

The family crisis interview with the potentially resistant family begins with the therapist politely asking the designated spokesperson what the presenting problem is. Usually, the best phrase is simply "What brings you here today?" After the spokesperson has been "consulted," input is obtained from the rest of the family. As a general rule of thumb, we have found it useful to spend approximately half of the first ten minutes in the session with the spokesperson talking, and half with the rest of the family. In our clinical work we have found it matters very little if family members are spoken to separately or together during this first phase.

Occasionally, pertinent information may arise during personal interviews, most often from children (e.g., from a six-year-old child who accompanied her mother and stepfather into an emergency assessment for depression: "Ralph makes Mommy dress up in funny clothes and walk up the street to make new boyfriends and then I get scared"). If the emergency therapist suspects incest or physical abuse as a possibility, greater care should be taken to interview each adult and child separately.

However, after the therapist has gained some rapport and generated at least a working hypothesis regarding the cause of the crisis, the therapist should insist that the family be interviewed together.

Ventilation

Frequently with the resistant family, the spokesperson, or some other important family figure, seeks prolonged discourse regarding one or more issues concerning the IP. This conversation is often peppered with accounts of how long-suffering the spokesperson has been, or descriptions of various sacrifices family members have made for the IP. Novice family therapists frequently allow excessive ventilation which not only consumes time but increases family enmity.

Some ventilation regarding the crisis is appropriate, inasmuch as it fosters empathy and rapport between the client family and the therapist. For example, ventilation may be necessary following instrumental stressors, such as when a family member has witnessed a terrible accident or experienced a significant trauma. Usually, however, it is more helpful for the therapist to move beyond ventilation in an attempt to directly influence the emotional climate of the family. Some useful techniques are discussed below.

Ventilation is frequently used by family members as an ineffectual means of attempting to punish or humiliate the IP. While "testimonials" of this type may be useful in longer-term family therapy, they are not usually productive during emergencies. They are also another method of dysfunctional coping. Unfortunately, the popular perception of crisis intervention is that it allows unlimited and unrestricted opportunities for the alleged "victim" to ventilate. This perception may be reinforced if the would-be-ventilator is accustomed to calling client-centered crisis lines that allow and encourage the caller to talk in an unbridled fashion. Persons who receive family-oriented crisis intervention may respond with anger at the therapist when they do not receive the opportunity to be heard to their satisfaction. High risk families may even ritualize professional crisis intervention as a means of punishing the IP in a public forum. Case Study 6.1, below, illustrates this.

Family Study 6.1. Jean and Bob

Jean was a successful oncologist. Somewhat shy and socially awkward, she was devastated when her husband left her for another woman. Jean routinely worked 50 to 60 hours a week. She also attempted to balance her occupational demands with the family responsibilities associated with raising two children from a first marriage.

Bob was a successful divorced attorney who met Jean while he was obtaining a deposition. He claimed that it was "love at first sight" and began courting her incessantly. The couple was married after a brief period of dating. Almost from their first week of marriage they displayed severe conflicts. Bob expected Jean to fulfil the role of traditional wife, including cooking meals and always being home after his long work days. He was angry at her inability to meet these needs, although felt ashamed to discuss his seemingly irrational desires to Jean. Consequently, the couple's home life was tense and periodically explosive.

Because he felt increasingly frustrated with his home life, Bob sought professional help from a local psychologist. His therapist encouraged him to ventilate his feelings in weekly individual therapy. This treatment had little effect and Bob began calling the local crisis line whenever he was frustrated with his spouse.

After several months, Bob's calls to the crisis line became routine. He would call every Wednesday, when he ordinarily got home several hours before Jean. He would ventilate a long list of purported wrongs, occasionally sounding somewhat paranoid.

On Saturdays, when Jean worked all day at the hospital, Bob would go to the local tavern. He would "hold court" in a section of the bar humorously reserved for "unwed husbands," men of higher socioeconomic status in the same position as Bob. While most of the other husbands seemed to enjoy this time away from home, Bob appeared distraught. He would constantly reiterate about how he had been "ripped off" by marrying Jean and how he wished he could "go home to a little homebody." Saturday evenings, after watching sports all day at the bar, Bob would return home drunk and verbally abuse Jean and her children.

Because Jean felt genuinely guilty about her time away from the family, she would patiently allow Bob to continue his irrational tirades. Bob would eventually pass out. Jean would then feel bad about herself. This pattern continued for several years.

Couples like Bob and Jean often are highly resistant to defusion during the initial family interview. Upon entering couples therapy they attempted to repeat their previous patterns to their new therapist. Bob came to the first session with a list of "demands" necessary to preserve the marriage. He tried to use the first session to align with the therapist against his wife. He became volatile when the therapist would not meet his agenda for the session.

When someone in the first–or any subsequent–family session attempts to present an agenda based on the need for ventilation, it is often best to encourage them to write about their feelings rather than bringing them up in the session. We encourage such clients to keep a journal at home, and perhaps to mail it to the therapist rather than to bring up its contents in the therapy session. The therapist can read these writings at a later date outside of the session. The client's anger is usually mollified and the therapy session can proceed to address more substantial issues. As tension in the family decreases the need for journaling declines. Other uses of therapeutic writing are available in the book by L'Abate (1992), and are useful in a number of therapeutic situations.

Tension Reduction

A helpful framework for any type of therapist work is the realization that crisis interviews are acutely stressful. They produce tension and this stress is two-sided. If the therapist feels anxiety when facing a potentially unmanageable situation, imagine what the client family feels!

Accordingly, L'Abate (1986) states that the first session in family therapy should be designed to reduce acute stress and build trust. Haley (1976) also comments on the importance of the first interview for instilling trust and providing a working alliance. A major step in working with high risk families in acute crisis is to reduce their tension levels so that subsequent work can proceed.

Acute tension can be reduced through a number of methods. Pittman (1987) discusses the potential desirability of pharmacological intervention for family members and generally discounts their use. He states pithily, "I've found that Haydn chamber music, popcorn, or an air of confidence calms everyone down almost as well as locking someone up" or providing medication (p. 32). However, medication is sometimes necessary for defusion and the nonmedical crisis specialist should always have collaborative access to a physician colleague.

Therapists who act with appropriate poise are the ones who are most effective in controlling crisis tension. The ineffable role of the therapist's confidence in his or her own abilities is one of the hardest aspects of family crisis intervention to teach. It is also difficult to measure and evaluate. More than likely, the reduction in time that experienced family crisis therapists are able to display when intervening in family systems is due to the superior confidence these therapists have in their own abilities. Families seem to respond affirmatively to this with a reduction in acute tension.

When family stress is extreme, it is often appropriate for the therapist to use brief relaxation exercises to reduce the stress level. The therapist must accompany these, or any other intervention, with a gentle and reassuring voice that indicates he or she is in control of the situation. Some therapists find visualization techniques useful for reducing extreme stresses. Others find an office with relatively low lighting of use (Pittman, 1987).

In severe cases, the therapist may find it necessary or useful to put the whole family under a hypnotic trance or pseudo trance. The following is an example of the use of some techniques in the very early stages of a crisis interview that can help decrease stress and increase trust.

Family Study 6.2. The "L" Family

Louisa is a 29-year-old lawyer who lives with her parents in her childhood home. She has never left home, having attended college and law school locally. Also present are both parents and an older sister. The parents are first generation immigrants in failing health. Louisa has telephoned the therapist asking for advice how to leave her aging parents. She recently has started dating for the first time in her life and wants to spend time alone with her boyfriend. According to Louisa, her mother told her boyfriend that she was dating someone else, apparently sabotaging her current relationship "so I wouldn't leave home." On the telephone, Louisa was calm and relaxed. She readily agreed to bring the "available family" in. However, in the office Louisa appears frustrated and labile.

Therapist: Now what seems to be the problem?

Louisa: It's just, oh, God, I never (laughing), never thought I'd being seeing . . . a shrink!

Therapist: Many people are initially uncomfortable. But, most people find it helpful.

Louisa: It's just that . . . it's just that (affect changes) I am so angry at my parents. I am so goddamn angry at them. I am furious at them, I am so goddamn angry at them. I am so angry at them for what they did that I can't even . . . I can't even . . . I can't even think about it.

Therapist: Hmmm. Okay, I want you to breathe deeply. That's right, a deep breath, very slowly. Now, I want you to count to ten as you breathe deeply. Okay, (with client) One, two . . . ten. Now, Now that we're relaxed, I want you to tell me what the problem seems to be at this time.

Louisa: Okay, okay, (subdued). I guess the problem is I'm 29 years old and I want to move out. But I feel guilty if I think about it. And I feel they don't want to let me go and will sabotage anything I do.

Mrs. L (mother): Oh, that's a lie. Another lie. You'll have to forgive my daughter. Ever since she was a small girl, she lies. She confuses things. She does not mean to. She just gets the facts mixed up.

Louisa: Oh, Mother, stop. Just be quiet. She always does this, talks for me. She . . .

Mr. L. (Interrupting): Someone has to talk for you. You are only a young woman. Not even married. No husband to talk for you. That's why the good Lord gave you parents.

Louisa: Goddamn it, stop talking for me!

Mrs. L.: Such language! You see, Doctor, I told you, she gets nervous and confuses things.

Louisa (to therapist): Now can you see? Can you see the nightmare I live with! No wonder I'm a going crazy . . .

Therapist: I think we *all* need to relax here. Now everyone, *slowly*. Count to ten. Breathe deeply. And then, and then (very subdued), I want you to remember, a happy scene. It doesn't have to be anything recent. I want you to sit back, slowly recall it, remember every detail and how it made you feel . . . . Close your eyes, and keep thinking . . . . Now, when I tell you to, I want you to open your eyes. You will feel relaxed and you will be able to talk without yelling at each other.

Some therapists might have encouraged the family to attack one another for a few more minutes to gain a picture of present functioning and communication skills. Therapists who do this often equate anger with candor. Perhaps this is true and of some value. However, this is not recommended for the early stages of the interview when little is known regarding the family's functioning, stress level, capacity for stress, or reason for presentation.

In this transcript, the therapist used both individual breathing relaxation, and a group relaxation technique that borders on hypnosis. In some cases, clients are suspicious of these techniques, especially if they hold stigmatized views of therapy or have had prior unsatisfactory experience with hypnosis. The therapist should be clear in his purpose and explain it to the family as follows:

> *Therapist:* Good. Now this exercise is often helpful in getting people to relax so that we can talk more openly. Remember (very slowly) our only goal is to talk more freely.

Occasionally, as in this case, family members will directly question whether they are being placed in a trance-like state. There are numerous public and professional misconceptions regarding hypnotism. Some people believe they will lose their minds or become pawns of the therapist. Individuals of some religious orientations believe that hypnotism is "Satanic," "of the Devil," or similar to necromancy. The term "deep relaxation," is a technically equivalent synonym without pejorative connotations.

Reframing

Many family therapists advocate reframing of the crisis to reduce its impact and hence to defuse it (e.g., Haley, 1976; L'Abate, 1986). Clearly, reframing can produce dramatic results in its ability to defuse a crisis, especially for resistant families. In many circumstances, reframing is a potent intervention. However, such families may have also heard various reframings before and grown cynical regarding their viability. The family study below illustrates this tendency.

Family Study 6.3. The O'Shaunasys

> As an example of the difficulty in using reframing methods to defuse crises, we recall our failure with the case of Robert O'Shaunasy, a young man of 19 with a history of numerous hospitalizations for acute alcohol intoxication. To the many therapists who had been involved in this case over the past five years, Robert's drinking pattern was clearly apparent: when Robert's mother and father began to move their disputes from the bedroom into the living room, Robert would begin drink-

ing to distract attention away from the marital dyad. At this point, Mrs. O'Shaunasy would cease haranguing her husband and concentrate instead upon getting her son into a state facility. Mr. O'Shaunasy would also join in the efforts, dutifully contacting his elected representatives, seeing if they could manipulate the long wait list for public assisted substance abuse inpatient services.

Once in the hospital, the family would rally around their son with unusual displays of warmth, empathy, and kindness. However, whenever the inpatient staff would suggest that the parents' difficulties related to their son's drinking, Robert would sign out, usually within a day or two.

The crisis therapist who answered Mrs. O'Shaunasy's call agreed to interview the family for pre-screening regarding hospitalization. There were no state beds available, and none would be open for several days. The therapist, an extremely seasoned social worker, tried to defuse the crisis somewhat by gently suggesting that Robert might drink because it brought the family closer together.

Mrs. O'Shaunasy became livid at this suggestion. "What kind of quack are you?" the mother screamed. "I've gone through this thing (the cycle of her son's binge drinking) twenty times. Each time, I've busted my ass trying to save my son. Any idiot knows he drinks because he has his father's Irish genes. I ought to report you for an ethical violation, because of your stupidity!"

Our guidelines for working with reframing are that techniques must be tempered with clinical experience and a sensitivity to the family's receptiveness. If the family does not endorse the reframing, the intervention may be used as an excuse to terminate ongoing therapy. Unless the reframing is immediately endorsed by one or more family members, its acceptance should probably not be compelled. In such cases, the "reframing failure" should be presented to the family as merely one of several hypotheses that might be applicable to their present difficulty. It is almost never helpful to insist upon a single view of the resistant family's problems that is contrary to the family's conception. On the other hand, if the family endorses the reframing it may be a valuable tool in helping them cope more functionally.

The Risks of Defusing a System

Healthy families regulate their behaviors in order to maintain a state of equilibrium that allows them to adjust to daily situations, including occasional crises or normal difficulties encountered by every family on a day-to-day basis. Resistant families are less capable of making these necessary homeostatic fine-tunings. A prototype similar to a hydraulic model is often invoked to describe resistant families and their response to stress. Periodically, pressure builds and the system needs a safety valve to open and relieve that pressure. The crisis provides this escape, and the system returns to more or less normal functioning. Again, this is an example of dysfunctional coping.

Providing crisis defusion is not without risks. Previously we indicated that individuals or families whose needs are not met during crisis intervention often go elsewhere. This is not surprising, since crises frequently have positive (but temporary) homeostatic significance for the family. Systems that are prematurely defused will often report that they have been "cured" or otherwise greatly helped by the interventions they have received. Often, these families are some of the most gratifying systems to work with–at least temporarily. Yet they will return to crisis, sometimes in a matter of hours.

Our task as clinicians is to defuse a crisis without devoiding it of its emotionality or systemic functioning for the family experiencing it. This is not an easy task. A general principle many clinicians have found useful is to initially assume that the family crisis–especially the perceptual crisis–has a functional or homeostatic value for one or more family members. The *art* of family-oriented crisis intervention involves knowing how to defuse and not destroy the functionality of the crisis for the family.

Learning the art of defusing a crisis while not *prematurely* defusing it is one of the most difficult aspects of crisis-oriented family therapy training. Essentially, however, the novice therapist does well if he or she treats the client's system crisis with respect, dignity, and seriousness, regardless of how inconsequential the crisis appears to be. This may be difficult inasmuch as trivial and sometimes comical perceptual crises may assume tremendous importance with resistant families. Yet, despite the objective seriousness–or lack of seriousness–we treat the crisis as a method of the family system that is attempting to maintain homeostasis. Our goal is to decrease the need for a crisis to provide the necessary homeostasis by empowering the family toward more functional coping. Directly or indirectly discounting a family's symptoms will encourage them to return in a greater state of dysfunction. Again, we must reiterate, even the craziest of families must be treated with respect and dignity.

One clue for unraveling the value of the crisis upon the family system's functioning is to look for the amount of exaggeration of symptomatology that is present during the family interview. Prior to assembling the family, the therapist may have heard various accounts of the IP's behavior from diverse family members. Often, when the therapist is trying to defuse the system, it will become clear that these accounts are grossly exaggerated. In general, the more exaggerated the symptoms and the longer they remain exaggerated, the more value the family system places upon the crisis as a means of restoring the homeostatic mechanisms of the family system. Why this is true remains unclear and, admittedly, we have no data to support this observation. Yet clinical experience has suggested this to be a convenient measure of the value that the family places on the crisis to restore systemic functioning.

Exaggeration of symptoms by family members tends to peak during the first half hour of the session. Furthermore, as the crisis interview continues, the number of symptom exaggerators in the family system begin to decrease. It is usually not necessary to confront wild or bizarre symptom exaggeration when it occurs, since it almost invariably "winds down" of its own. However, if exaggeration continues, or when the accounts of one family member are grossly incongruent with those of others in the system, the careful therapist must ask him or herself "What is going on?" Almost always, systems that continue to exaggerate the behavior of the IP are systems in desperate trouble, begging for a respite. Unless the exaggerated accounts are originating from family members who are psychotic, extreme care needs to be taken in these cases. Often, such systems will go elsewhere to meet their enormous needs. And, if this fails, the system may increase it symptomatology, with the IP or other family members typically becoming more resistant and deviant.

An example of this phenomena is often encountered regarding hospitalization of family members. In the days of generous inpatient mental health insurance coverage in the United States, it was quite common for families to succeed in hospitalizing IPs at the smallest suggestion of family disharmony. This provided a convenient way for families to scapegoat members and avoid the painful process of examining their collective behavioral sequences. Fortunately, this is rather rare today, as it has become more difficult to involuntarily hospitalize someone.

However, some families have learned they may increase the chances of hospitalization by magnifying the lethality of the IP's behavior. This may occur consciously or unconsciously. Whereas a generation ago, a brief psychotic reaction to a family quarrel would guarantee hospitalization of the IP, now, the stakes have to be increased to get beyond the hospital door, especially if the patient is indigent or if insurance benefits have been exhausted. In some cases the family will exaggerate the IP's behavior to emergency workers performing mental health screening. More often, however, both the patient and the family learn the unwritten rules and act accordingly. These rules may involve the patient's temporary decompensation whenever the family needs a "breather." When the therapist chooses to disregard these rules there is the possibility the family will worsen, rather than improve. This is tragically illustrated in the high risk family below:

Family Study 6.4. The Ciccecci Family

Anthony was a 39-year-old chronic schizophrenic who had been hospitalized seven times since his first break at 17. He lived in an isolated rural area with his mother, 62, a former nurse and father, 71, a retired accountant. Anthony was extremely unkempt, chain-smoking and drinking soft drinks constantly. His mother believed that he needed constant supervision. She stated that she was frequently "exhausted" by caring for him. Anthony's older sister was killed in a car accident. A younger brother, Bob, 36, is a science fiction writer who lives several hours away. Anthony's father is showing early signs of dementia and is occasionally combative.

About once a year, Anthony's mother claimed that Anthony threatened to overdose or slit his wrists. When questioned, Anthony denied these allegations, stating that his mother was the one that was "schizo." Bob noted that this behavioral pattern usually followed a period of prolonged family tension. Anthony would then be driven to the local emergency room, and then to the state hospital 90 miles away. He always managed to sign in with voluntary status. Bob stated that his mother appeared happier during these hospitalizations. Bob also believed that the unwritten family rule was that the mother would relinquish care of Anthony for this period, with Bob taking on the role of daily hospital visitor to his brother. According to Bob, "When Anthony was in the hospital Mom did things she would never think of doing otherwise. Like going to church, going shopping for herself, and getting her hair done. After about three weeks of this, she felt guilty and took him out against medical advice. Sometimes the staff took it to court, but usually they didn't bother."

The family treatment of patients like Anthony illustrates some difficulties regarding hospitalization with resistant families. Before deinsitutionalization, Anthony would have been hospitalized for years. Presumably, the family system would not have evolved to care for him. The therapist may be tempted to wink at the familial pattern, and allow the family system to meet its needs with regularity by tacitly condoning these brief hospitalizations. After all, the family does deserve some respite, even if their coping mechanism is clearly dysfunctional.

On the other hand, the therapist might attempt a number of interventions designed to keep Anthony out of the hospital. These include increasing medication and reducing psychosocial stressors. However, if Anthony is responding to a system that needs to hospitalize him in order to restore itself, then it is likely that Anthony will act crazier when brief interventions are attempted and are initially successful. The symptoms of persons such as these must be given initial credence to the family and the functional value of the family's behavior must be supplanted with more effective coping tasks.

When this does not occur the results can be tragic. Anthony was refused hospital admission on five consecutive occasions because the emergency worker prescreening him believed his symptoms could be managed at home. The worker recommended a variety of interventions designed to reduce the necessity for hospitalization and to decrease family tension. These worked well. However, the worker failed to understand that Anthony's symptoms continued to increase with each "successful" intervention. A few days later Anthony asphyxiated after ingesting an overdose of psychotropic medication. Had the emergency worker attended more to the functional value of Anthony's symptoms for the family, she might have acted differently and Anthony might still be alive.

How do we know if we have inadvertently "smothered" a family's problems, rather than adequately defusing them? One indication is when the family suddenly becomes *too* compliant during the initial interview. Acquiescence is usually a sign that the family is disregarding whatever intervention is being proposed. Or, a previously active family may become silent and taciturn. All of these are warning signs that a family is resisting. Similarly, families that abruptly halt their symptom exaggeration have probably been defused too quickly. When these things occur in the crisis session the best course is to allow family members to ventilate just a bit in order to increase the family tension. This is one of the few instances where we believe it is appropriate to increase tension during an initial interview. Again, the problem is attempting to balance this increase in family tension with the need to defuse the system. Unfortunately, there are no hard rules and clinical experience and judgement are important, as usual.

FAMILY CRISIS EVALUATION (E): THE FRAMEWORK FOR EMPOWERMENT

After a crisis has been sufficiently defused so that the participants can communicate concerns, the therapist immediately begins the process of evaluating the family. Evaluation includes five major components. First, the family is evaluated for traditional psychiatric concerns, such as homicidal and suicidal ideation, and ability of family members to care for themselves. Secondly, the family crisis is appraised for the degree of crisis instrumentality. Third, the family is then evaluated for their status as a high risk–i.e., a crisis-prone and treatment resistant system. Fourth, family coping styles are assessed. Finally, potential family and external resources are estimated. During the entire procedure, the therapist is formulating a plan to attempt to manage the family's crisis in a manner that will encourage them to solve their own problems, without reliance on dysfunctional coping. Each of these portions of the family assessment will be discussed below.

Traditional Psychiatric Assessment

Family intervention with resistant systems cannot ignore traditional psychiatric nomenclature. Nor can it overlook the fundamentals of the traditional mental status examination. These include determining whether clients are hallucinating, or oriented to person, place, and time. They also involve assessing the homicidal and suicidal ideation of the IP and also of other potentially problematic family members. Finally, they involve assessing whether or not the IP and others in the family can adequately care for themselves.

It is incumbent upon the family crisis therapist to be able to perform competent diagnoses and assessment of these areas. Because of this we strongly encourage family therapists to obtain substantial inpatient experience, or at least exposure to clients whose mental status warrants hospitalization. In our opinion, there is no substitution for this experience that can teach the uses–and abuses–of psychiatric hospitalization.

Almost every mental health professional is well versed in the statutory and common law requirements regarding duty to warn significant others of potential danger from a client. Equally clear and well known are requirements involving breach of confidentiality for child and elder abuse and neglect. These will not be reviewed here since they vary according to jurisdictions. However, as McCown and Johnson (1991) have indicated, incest and child abuse are relatively common in resistant families. Clinicians should always keep this possibility in mind.

The possibility of liability in family crisis intervention is potentially magnified when more than one family member is seen. For example, we are aware of a case where the son was brought in for evaluation and a week later the husband attempted suicide. Fortunately for the therapist, in this case there was no litigation. It remains to be seen whether courts will hold family therapists liable for negligence when a family member other than the IP harms self or another. Because of this possibility we routinely document the mental status of each member of the family system that is present, whether or not they are an "open case."

Assessment for Crisis Instrumentality

It is possible and sometimes common to interview a resistant family for several hours and to miss the fact that they have no place to sleep or nothing to eat. Sometimes families simply forget to mention extremely critical information. Individuals and especially families in crisis frequently lose perspective of time. They may intend to tell the therapist crucial data, but simply lose track of the clock.

Families may also attempt to conceal unfavorable information until the end of the interview. They may do this because they want the therapist to like and respect them. This commonly occurs following an Instrumental Crisis. Medical emergency room personnel encounter this phenomena frequently. For instance, a spouse might give a complete and exhaustive medical history to an E.R. nurse, and then comment sheepishly, at the logical conclusion of the interview, "One other thing I think you might need to know. I said Harry doesn't usually drink, and I mean that. He's a good Christian. But he has been drunk for the last ten days."

Sometimes families are simply too numbed from an Instrumental crisis to request assistance. This is illustrated below.

Family Study 6.5. The Olmsteads

The Olmsteads were inland victims of Hurricane Hugo's unexpected devastation a hundred miles from the South Carolina coast. Their house was completely leveled and they had no source of food or shelter. When interviewed by a crisis worker, the family appeared rather indifferent to their plight. Mr. Olmstead stated that he would "just find something, somewhere." Mrs. Olmstead stated that "We can always stay with neighbors," despite the fact that neighbors had almost all experienced similar devastating losses. The only concern of note in the family was that expressed by Janey, age eight, who was worried that she would have to be separated from her pet cat.

The therapist who was "triaging" this case made a note of the family's imminent needs and sought to link the family to appropriate social and crisis-oriented services.

We have found a simple list of questions extremely helpful in assisting families who may potentially be undergoing an Instrumental Crisis. Not all are relevant for each family, and not all need to be asked. However, the therapist should have the answers to all of these at least by the midpoint of the clinical interview's allotted time. See Table 6.1 for a list of these questions.

TABLE 6.1. Instrumental Questions

1. Where is the family staying?
2. Is anyone in the family in danger?
3. Do you have enough to eat?
4. What are your plans tomorrow?
5. Is anyone in the family ill?
6. Is anyone in the family acting irrationally?
7. Are there other family members who aren't present who may have problems?
8. Do you know who to contact in an emergency?
9. Are you worried about the health or safety of anyone in the family?
10. Is there any reason to suspect that any of this information might change soon?

For families that are having difficulty functioning, it may be necessary for the therapist to ask these questions directly and repeatedly, though with sensitivity.

We stress that these questions should be answered relatively early in the interview. It is not uncommon for families to "drop a bomb" at the end of the session by announcing that they "just remembered, we don't have any place to go tonight and we're out of money." Therapists typically make the inference that these "bombs" are manipulative. Within the context an Instrumental Crisis, however, they are more than likely due to a genuine failure by the family to adequately assess and recall present circumstances. For example, a tourist family that is in shock over being robbed may not recall until the close of the interview that their assailants took their hotel money, credit cards, and car keys.

Evaluation of Crisis-Proneness and Treatment Resistance

It is usually easy to determine how crisis-prone a family system is. Simply ask. Most clients answer honestly when they are asked, "Does your family have many crises?" Clients who are too hostile or uncooperative to answer this question usually need more crisis delusion.

To maintain a higher degree of accuracy, we prefer to base our assessment on the answer provided by the family spokesperson. The specific terminology used in phrasing the question is not as important as the family's understanding that the therapist is interested in problems that occurred during the previous twelve months. The family amy occasionally ask, "What do you mean by a crisis?" to which the therapist should respond, "When things felt like they were outside of the control of you or your family."

The number of crises can be charted on a number line or included as clinical notes. The one month reliability of this method with the family spokesperson is acceptable, though not outstanding (.59). The reliability is certainly attenuated by the fact that when people are in crisis their judgment regarding past crises is changed, and probably, due to the phenomenon of state dependent learning, their memories are enhanced. Family members disagree considerably regarding how many crises the family has been in during the previous year, with a negative correlation between the recollection of the family spokesperson and the IP (−.11). While neither may necessarily be more accurate than the other, our approach has found it useful to accept the account of the spokesperson for basing our assessment on how crisis-prone the family system really is.

Determining treatment resistance is another matter altogether. In fortuitous circumstances the therapist will have clinical records or anecdotal accounts available and will be able to estimate the likelihood that the family will resist treatment recommendations. When this information is not accessible, it is important that the therapist surmise these details. Although we are often tempted to directly ask "How many times have you dropped out of treatment during the past year?" such questions are both offensive to the family and useless. More subtle phraseology must be employed.

Often effective is the empathetic inquiry regarding the frequency that the family has felt "at the brink" during the past year and what they have done to "regroup." Families can then be queried regarding what they did to solve their past crises. This furnishes extremely valuable information regarding the family's high risk status. Family Study 6.6 below illustrates some of the useful phrases clinicians may employ to elicit this information. This study is also presented because the family continually frustrated the therapist's initial attempts to gather this information, resulting in her use of a number of phrases that usually by themselves are able to solicit the needed information.

Family Study 6.6. The Caravelle Family

The family, Mr. Caravelle, age 54, and his wife, age 49, presented to an emergency room with Mrs. Caravelle's 79-year-old mother, Mrs. McGinnis. According to Mr. Caravelle, Mrs. McGinnis has been "acting crazy" and "needs to get into the hospital." However, upon interview, the mother, Mrs. McGinnis, is polite, fully oriented, and appropriate.

Therapist: How that we've all had time to discuss what brought us here, I'm' going to shift gears a little bit. I'm wondering how often recently–say in the past year or so–you have felt like you've had the last straw.

Mr. C.: I don't know. I don't think about those things.

Therapist: And you, Mrs. Caravelle?

Mrs. C.: I don't know, either. Maybe a lot. Maybe a little. What's it to you?

Mr. C.: I tell you what it is to her. She wants to send us home with your mother after patting us on the back. Telling us we're doing a good job and that kind of bullshit.

Therapist: Whoa! We're ahead of ourselves! I'm just trying to figure out how much stress you all have been under. It sounds like things have been pretty hard at home.

Mr. C.: Maybe a lot. I don't know. I don't think like you shrinks. Stress, what is stress? I do my job. I go home. I want some peace. And now, we've got this crazy lady screaming and hollering, messing up our lives.

Mrs. M.: (oblivious to Mr. C.) Who knows? They fight all the time, mostly about money. Lordy, you should see them fight!

Mrs. C.: Shut up, Mother.

Mrs. M.: It's true. They fight all the time. And then they're mean to me (bursts into tears). Then they hit me. They hit me.

Mr. C.: She's lying. She's crazy. That's why we need to have her put in the hospital.

Therapist: I'm sure it must have been difficult, living with an elderly person the past year.

Mr. C.: Goddamn right!

Therapist: You've probably wanted to do it many times before . . .

Mrs. C.: But this time it's serious. I'm telling you.

Therapist: What's kept you from trying to get her into the hospital before?

Mr. C.: What's kept us? Hell, we've tried a half dozen times. Each time they tell us no, that we're not eligible or something like that.

Therapist: Hmmm (incredulously). Not eligible?

Mr. C.: Yeah, they say take her home for a while and she'll get better. I'm telling you, she hasn't gotten better. Does she look better? They tell us to do all this, you know, take her to the elderly center during the day and shit like that. Like I have time? Like the wife has time? Gimme a break! I say she needs to be put away. Stop driving me crazy.

Assessing treatment resistant proneness is more subjective than crisis-proneness. We use a seven-point scale for ratings. Higher numbers are associated with a greater likelihood of resistance. The seven categories that we use are described below.

1. *Motivated families in crisis that have no or almost no treatment experience.* These families should be treated as if they are completely treatment compliant. Over 95 percent of such families return for future therapy.

2. *Motivated families in crisis that have a history of successful treatment.* Such are compliant to treatment most of the time. However, in about 20 percent of these cases they may be noncompliant, as indicated by abrupt terminations and missed sessions. Sometimes this is because they are momentarily discouraged. They feel that since they were "cured once" they should be problem free, or they may not like their crisis therapist, or his or her modality, and prefer the previous therapist.

3. *Families in crisis that are presently involved in unsuccessful, or only moderately successful treatment.* These families remain convinced, on at least some level, that they can solve their problem. These families have not given up hope. They are motivated to change, yet confused about the process. Since these families are usually referred back to their therapists, the percentage of noncompliance is unknown.

4. *Families in crisis that have terminated unsuccessful treatment one or more times, yet are seeking additional intervention from professionals.* These families are the "desperate" families clinicians often see. They may be cynical regarding the possibility for change but they have a flicker of hope. If engaged carefully, they

may prove treatment compliant. However, they are uncompliant at least one-third of the time.

5. *Families in crisis that are nihilistic or fatalistic about their problems and believe that nothing will work.* They may have "tried it all." They feel despair and a sense of desperateness. Similarly, they may believe their problems are due to biology or other factors that cannot be changed. These families are compliant less than half of the time.

6. *The family in crisis that feels their therapeutic failures prove they are more competent than mental health professionals and can manage their own systems better than professionals.* In general, we believe that this is a positive sign of mental health. Yet when they are crisis-prone this obviously is not true. Often, families of this type are "service shopping" as described in Chapter One. They want a specific intervention, and often want the therapist to fix their family immediately. If they do not get this service they may go elsewhere. Our data suggest that about 70 percent of these families will not comply with our recommendations.

7. *The family in crisis that is composed primarily of members who are unaware of the dysfunctional aspects of their situation or recurrent behaviors, e.g., a mother and father who are both severe schizophrenics.* These families may not see the need to keep their children adequately clothed. Another example might be a family of Satanists who encourage their children to sacrifice neighborhood pets as part of their religious rituals. Families that are this severely impaired are often labeled as deviant and have usually been involved with many social service systems. They are also invariably treatment resistant. They are compliant less than 15 percent of the time.

The information gained regarding crisis-proneness and especially treatment resistance is employed to determine appropriate interventions, discussed in the next chapter. Usually the information can be gained by strategically or indirectly asking about previous treatment experiences and failures. When it appears that the family may have had multiple treatment failures, the therapist can innocently ask something like this: "It sounds like you have had a lot of experience in the mental health field. What kind of approach would you recommend for people who have your sorts of problems?" This question reframes the family's experience from being "losers" to "educated consumers." The therapist may wish to embellish these phrases further for families that seem to disdain mental health professionals.

An excellent example of this use of indirect querying that also empowers a treatment resistant family is shown in the transcript below.

Family Study 6.7. The Sloanes

> John and Maria Sloane, 43 and 45, sought crisis therapy regarding their chronic schizophrenic son, Jonathan. From the beginning it was evident that the couple wanted to disagree with everything the therapist said. The couple also seemed to enjoy disagreeing with each other. The therapist was able to use both traits to his advantage and gain otherwise unobtainable information.
>
> *Therapist:* And what about help for Jonathan in the past? I'm sorry, but I don't have a clear picture yet.
>
> *John:* We've tried everything. Like I told you. Nothing works.
>
> *Maria:* Nothing. No sense in going over them all. I told you, nothing was any value with Jonathan.
>
> *Therapist:* Hmm. Well, if things are as hopeless as they seem, I mean as serious as they seem, maybe I could use you to help me, at least. I'll be honest with you. There is a lot of fluff–maybe even frauds–in this field. People do–promise, yeah, promise all kinds of things that are just impossible. I was wondering if you could tell me about some of your therapy experiences that were the least helpful. I mean, maybe even when you got ripped off or something.
>
> *Maria:* (Laughs) You want *all* of them! We'd be here all day. Let's see . . .
>
> At this point the couple rudely competed with each other to see who could provide the most detailed history of Jonathan's

treatment. On the basis of this it became evident that Jonathan had never been tried for a sufficient length of time on an antipsychotic medication.

Therapist ratings of family treatment resistance are not perfectly reliable, though surprisingly they are higher than the reliability of crisis-proneness ratings. Our data indicate that the interrater reliability for ratings is about .74, which, while not outstanding, is probably acceptable for clinical work. We have considered adding various weighted questions to our seven-point scale such as adding one point to the scale if the family's problem has extended for more than a year. However, the simple but crude technique used here seems helpful enough. We have also experimented with assessment of resistance through various empirically derived and theory based questionnaires. Although we were able to obtain a much higher degree of reliability with psychometrically adequate scales, the additional information is probably not worth the trade-off in effort and potential alienation of the family by invasive paperwork. Structured clinical assessment is adequate enough.

Assessing Dysfunctional Coping

Therapists often observe a family for weeks or months before they are able to comment regarding the family's dysfunctional coping styles. This is because these styles are not likely to be evoked unless there is a family crisis. Crises produce what is known in the psychological literature as "state dependent recall." This means that individuals who are not in crisis may have difficulty remembering what they do when they are operating under crisis conditions. Similarly, people who are in crisis may find it hard to remember routine occurrences or personal histories that are not connected with crisis situations.

For these reasons people in crisis are simultaneously both poor and excellent historians. They may not be able to remember the names of previous therapists or medications or places of employment. However, they can often recall what they did to solve their previous crises, and if something has worked for them, even temporarily, there is a good likelihood they will employ it again. Therefore, the best way to assess crisis coping is to ask people in crisis what they have done in the past.

Previously, we have introduced McCubbin and Figley's (1983) schema for dysfunctional family coping. During our interview process we like to answer the following questions regarding family coping that are based upon McCubbin and Figley's approach:

1. *Identification of the Stressor.* Is your family usually able to identify what is bothering it during a crisis?
2. *Locus of the Problem.* When there is a problem at home do people consider it a *family* problem or an individual problem?
3. *Approach to the Problem.* In the past, when there have been problems at home can your family try to solve them together?
4. *Tolerance of Others.* Does your family get along well with those outside of it? Neighbors? School officials? Employers?
5. *Commitment to and Affection for Family Members.* Do you feel people in the family care for each other when there is a crisis? Do they display it or talk about their affection?
6. *Communication Utilization.* When something is wrong at home can people talk about it? Or do they get silent and "sit on their problems?"
7. *Family Cohesion.* When something bad happens at home does your family stick together? Or do they go their separate ways?
8. *Family Roles.* Can people in your home be flexible when someone is sick, under stress, or has a problem? Can you give examples?
9. *Resource Utilization.* Are there people outside of your immediate family whom you turn to for help when there is a crisis at home? Can you name a few?
10. *Violence.* (This question must be asked to both spouses and all family members present). Is there more violence at home than you would like when things get stressful at home? To whom does it occur?
11. *Non-Prescription Drugs and Alcohol.* (This question must also be asked to both spouses and all family members present) Do people at home drink or use drugs when there is a lot

of stress at home? Is this a typical pattern? If the family is reluctant to answer questions in this domain, a screening tool may be administered to family members.

Generally, these questions can be incorporated into the early stages of the interview in an unobtrusive manner. We have also experimented with administering them in written form, either in a questionnaire or structured clinical interview format, both with positive results especially from middle-class families with a high degree of verbal skills.

Dysfunctional coping mechanisms are likely to be "snag points" (to use Frank Pittman's useful phrase) around which the family displays conflict. Once information is obtained regarding their prevalence, the therapist makes a note of them and incorporates them into the treatment plan or behavioral contract, discussed in the next chapter. A safe assumption is that families will return to the use of dysfunctional coping methods in a very short period of time, unless their systemic tension decreases. We attempt to construct a behavioral contract that de-emphasizes their occurrences. In this manner, other more functional homeostatic mechanisms are strengthened. Furthermore, the excessive homeostatic inclination which is the cause of family resistance is often weakened sufficiently so that longer-term treatment becomes an option rather than an impossibility.

Assessment for Abuse, Incest, and Violence

Possibly the most unique aspect of a family therapist's involvement with resistant families is the frequency with which the therapist must consider issues beyond the typical therapeutic contract. These include the issues of assessing and monitoring family systems that may be abusive to minors or disabled elderly, or where incest or domestic violence is prevalent. Therapists who confront these issues complain that they are more often called upon to play police officer or peacemaker than they are to conduct the actual work of therapy itself. When family therapists are called upon to step out of their typical role and take affirmative action to prevent abuse, a very real concern is the implications this has for their effectiveness as agents of meaningful systemic change. If the family system knows, for example, that they can manipulate the therapist by displays indicative of potential violence, the integrity of the therapist's stance is in jeopardy and, along with it, his or her capacity to affect the needed systemic changes. While this can occur in any family it is even more likely to occur in the treatment resistant system, which may be looking for any excuse at all to terminate therapy.

Although all therapists must struggle with the difficult issue of confidentiality and reporting requirements, the paradox is particularly difficult for a systems theorist working with resistant families. Not only must a family systems theorist struggle with the confidentiality issue, but he or she must also struggle with the ascription of legal consequences to a perpetrator who, in systems terms, is not solely to blame. The causal theory of child or elder abuse in systems terms is typically more systemic, circular, and diffuse. No singular individual is seen as the cause of the symptom. Consequently, when a family systems theorist is required to report an abusive parent or, in the cases of elderly persons, an abusive child or in-law, he or she feels not only the strain of breaking confidentiality, but also the implicit blaming of a perpetrator in a manner that runs contrary to the grain of her theoretical position.

In the context of clinical work, the literature makes it clear that the position of neutrality, adopted by some systems therapists as a part of a strategy to bring about change, must not be allowed to interfere with a primary, moral, and ethical responsibility to protect children from abuse (Asen et al., 1989; Boszormenyi-Nagy, 1985). Though substantial disagreement may exist in the literature as to the most appropriate causal model for understanding family violence or incest, it must be stressed that a systemic understanding of the problem should not be used as an excuse to ignore dangers of imminent harm to helpless child (or adult) victims. The only palatable conclusion at this point is for systems family therapists to swallow any theoretical contradiction implicit in reporting abusive situations and to then work with child welfare agencies to identify and implement the most appropriate short- and long-term solutions, some of which may involve non-separation under supervised conditions.

The secrecy and shame typically surrounding family violence often makes the assessment process a difficult one (Garbarino et al., 1986). The finding of abuse is somewhat less difficult in cases where the family has been referred for therapy due to a prior finding of abuse. Even in that situation, however, elicitation of the family dynamics surrounding the issue is still likely to be impeded by both shame and family expectations of privacy, as well as concern that the therapist's discoveries could be used to harm certain family members in court situations (Nichols, 1986).

To counteract the inclination to secrecy, as well as to obtain the most circumspect view of the problem as possible, the family therapist will most likely seek to interview each family member, including children. This is usually necessary, even in a crisis interview. Where the children are preverbal, or the material seems difficult to address with them, a play interview is often employed, in which children are asked to make up stories about dolls or to tell a story about the family. Through this less threatening approach, as well as some projective interpretation of the young child's speech, a therapist can often obtain a rich flavor of the family dynamics through the impressions the young child is developing of his or her interpersonal world (Garbarino et al., 1986).

Despite the inclination towards secrecy, the most common way of obtaining information from parents is through direct interview. Parents may be asked general questions regarding the present marital and child-related situation, the developmental history of the child and family, everyday activities, and general satisfaction with family life (Garbarino et al., 1986). Many authors suggest open-ended inquiries as a way of obtaining the necessary information without putting parents on guard by specific and threatening questions. In cases where a specific injury is observed, more direct questioning of both child and caretaker may be warranted.

Family history and the construction of a genogram may also yield substantial information about the dynamics of the present situation, although this information may be difficult to secure during emergency or crisis sessions. Discussion of whether a child was planned and wanted, the circumstances surrounding the birth, nursing practices, typical behaviors of the infant, and developmental milestones all may yield important factual information about the child's situation, as well as being a rich source of observation of the parent's affective connection and stance towards the child (Garbarino et al., 1986; Nichols, 1986).

The identification of a maltreated adolescent may often be easier than in the case of a younger child or infant because of the more extensive social network an adolescent likely possesses and the greater number of persons who likely possess information about the adolescent. Therefore, interviews with school counselors, teachers, peers, and friends are particularly useful for such evaluations. Behavioral manifestation of the maltreated adolescent may often take the form of truancy or running away, feelings of depression or worthlessness, somatic disturbances and even suicidal talk or gestures (Garbarino et al., 1986).

The adolescent assessment illustrates the general utility of our suggestion of involving as many sources of information as possible in all evaluations. Family doctors, pediatricians, school or day care personnel, and other professionals can provide information about family crises and adaptations that the family itself may be disinclined or even loathe to reveal. Garbarino et al. (1986) provide an extensive listing of family maltreatment assessment instruments, which may variously be filled out by the therapist, one or both of the parents, the children, or several combinations thereof, and which derive from several different theoretical orientations.

Particular issues of child and elder abuse with resistant families are so commonly encountered that we will devote additional chapters of this volume to them.

Assessment of Social Supports

The last major area we assess during our crisis intervention work is that of familial social support. As we indicated in Chapter Three in the discussion of the Hill/McCubbin model, resistant families are often satisfied with their social networks. Crisis prone families, on the other hand, often lack support. Typically, the clinician will want to inquire about a number of areas regarding the possibility of the family sharing their stressful burden with caring others.

Social support assessment can either be formal, with any number of excellent diagnostic instruments, or informal. Sometimes it is helpful to obtain information regarding social support from the family in a written form. Families can be asked to fill out a questionnaire regarding social support while they are in the waiting room or during the very first few minutes of a family session. Usually, families are quite cooperative regarding filling out such instruments, provided they are not lengthy.

In the case of informal assessment, the therapist should inquire about the following areas:

1. Where are the nearest *responsible* relatives that can assist the family?
2. Does the family have any close friends that may be of assistance during a crisis?
3. Can religious institutions be accessed, either for instrumental or spiritual support?
4. Is the family involved in any self-help groups that can be of aid during a crisis?

All of this information is vitally important. Some of our interventions may focus on ameliorating deficits in social supports. Often, it is more difficult to work these questions into the initial interview than it is to assess coping or even treatment history. Questions regarding social support may need to be queried directly if they are otherwise unanswered.

What We Do Not Assess in a Crisis Interview

There are a number of variables that may be related to family dysfunctioning that it might be useful to assess. For example, we would like to know how enmeshed a family is, the extent of triangling, how dependent or impulsive the family might be, and what sort of generational boundaries exist. We could also benefit further from having an accurate family history and genogram.

Unfortunately, obtaining this useful information from resistant families may be difficult and not feasible. From our research efforts we have found that resistant families fight both extraneous self-disclosure and the completion of clinical or research questionnaires. The longer the interview remains diagnostic, the less likely the family is to adhere to treatment recommendations or even to return for the next session.

Many times therapists can accurately assess family structural variables during the first session. However, sometimes they cannot do so and are completely wrong when they try. We suggest that unless there is substantial evidence otherwise, the clinician refrain from making significant inferences about the family's structural processes during the first interview. Exceptions to this general rule will be discussed later. Of course, if the family is well known to the therapist or adequate clinical records are available that document persistent structural problems within a family, then the therapist should unquestionably make use of this information during the problem-solving portion of the crisis interview.

There are certainly numerous assessment instruments that provide the family clinician with invaluable information. It is often tempting to administer them during the crisis interview. In our longer-term work we routinely use such tools as Olson, Portner, and Lavee's *FACES III* (1985), an instrument designed to assess a family's position on Olson's extraordinarily useful circumflex model. L'Abate (1986), among others, also has a number of worthwhile family assessment devices. But for our brief, problem-focused work we may be forced to do without this information. We do not want the family to use the excuse of "too much paperwork" as a reason to terminate. Furthermore, the literacy level required to complete many family inventories is quite high (Kaufman, Tarnowski, Simonian, & Graves, 1991). Too often we have embarrassed poorly educated families by our data collection. Not surprisingly, these families proved highly resistant.

Chapter Seven

Family Problem Solving: A Crisis Intervention/Consultation Approach

As we have indicated, the crisis interview with resistant families involves the therapist in progressive development as a systems *consultant* with reciprocal decrease in the role of traditional therapist. During the first three stages of the crisis session, Assembling, Defusement and Evaluation, the therapist primarily operates from a medical model, with the family viewed as acutely disturbed. The next stage, Problem Solving, represented by the letter P in our acronym, involves a gradual role transition with greater emphasis on facilitating the efforts of the family in problem identification and generation of solutions. During this stage the worker serves both as therapist and systems consultant to the family. This chapter will elucidate how we use this mixed therapeutic/consultational role to aid high risk families in solving their own problems.

DEVELOPING AND COMMUNICATING TENTATIVE CRISIS FORMULATIONS: THE FIRST STEP TOWARD FAMILY PROBLEM SOLVING

After defusion and evaluation it is often helpful for the crisis therapist/consultant–as we now label the crisis worker at this stage of the process–to provide a tentative formulation of difficulties for the family. Sometimes, the formulation is nothing more than affirmation by the therapist/consultant that the family does indeed have a serious problem requiring immediate attention. It is often beneficial if the therapist/consultant respectfully frames the problem as something that needs to be solved by the family *now*. "We" statements rather than more impersonal "You" statements often help to let the client family know they are being supported by the therapist/consultant. However, such statements become less appropriate in the final stages of the crisis session when the goal is empowerment of the family system to solve their own problems.

In addressing families we have found it useful for the therapist/consultant to apply the term "seems" regarding potential reasons for the problem at hand. An alternative phrase might be, "This is what is most likely the problem as it appears today." This is a stylistic technique popularized by students of Milton Erickson, who believe that such communications foment unconscious expectations that the problem will vary daily and in subjective causal attribution. In general, it is beneficial to maintain tentative formulations of problems, especially during crisis sessions. In short, we view family intervention as a process of hypothesis testing. Commitment to one hypothesis early in treatment may blind us to rival and more accurate hypotheses.

At this point in the process we begin to solicit the family's input and expertise regarding problem formulation. We often hypothesize one or more formulations to the family and ascertain whether they are reasonable or correct. It is beneficial to formulate the crisis problem on two levels: An immediate or precipitating problem and an overriding or precursor problem. These correspond to the notions of proximal and distal causes of crisis popular in social science literature.

Immediate problems include precipitating events that brought the family into crisis treatment. Families can often reach a consensus regarding such events, and the therapist/consultant may agree with the family (Perlmutter & Jones, 1985). However, individual views usually vary regarding culpability of family members in producing precipitating events. For example, most family members can reach an agreement that what prompted the present crisis was a discrete and specific event, such as Dad's drinking today, or Johnny stealing the car. They usually differ on determining who is to blame or why such behaviors occurred.

Precursor problems are more difficult to identify by the worker and harder to accept by the family. This contrasts with immediate problems, which are usually easily identifiable. One myth that resistant families often seem to endorse is that solution of all potential precipitating crises will enable the family to function smoothly forever. It is typical to hear the resistant family voice essentially unrealistic expectations such as "If only my husband would stop running around, we'd all be happy," or "If my son would simply quit drugs, everything would be fine."

It is not really necessary for the therapist to accurately diagnose a distal or precursor problem. Resistant families often have many problems. It is impossible to say with certainty which are causally related to the family's immediate plight. It is typically advantageous, however, for the worker to inform the family of the *possibility* that their problems contain more than surface issues. Sometimes this can be accomplished by directly telling the families there *might* be other problems that are present, but unnoticed. Often, the same goal can be realized by suggesting to families the tentativeness of their own problem formulation. It should be subtly stressed that their initial understanding and statement of the presenting problem is often not their final summation. Some useful techniques to meet this goal are presented in the family study below.

Family Study 7.1. The Gursons

Maureen and Steven Gurson, 21 and 23, sought emergency intervention from the local mental health center because Steven had been arrested for exposing himself in public. According to Steven this came about because he was drunk and he needed to urinate. Unfortunately, he happened to urinate in front of the store of an irate shopowner who called the police and pressed charges. Both Maureen and Steven believed that this was an isolated incident that would not reoccur. At this point in the transcript, the therapist/consultant is attempting to keep the couple open to the fact that they may have deeper problems than this mere civil infraction. He has attempted to assess Steven's drinking history, but with little success. The couple is openly hostile to each other and to the crisis worker, as well as guarded and mildly evasive. The therapist/consultant also suspects that they are somewhat sociopathic.

Therapist/consultant: As I see it, I guess the problem, on one level at least, is that Steven got caught and Maureen is angry.

Maureen: That's right. Of all the stupid . . .

Therapist/consultant: Hold on, remember our ground rule. No name-calling. Now Steven, what do you see as the problem?

Steven: So our problem is now they got me for exposure, which is a felony, as compared to urinating in public, which is a fine. Man, I'm going to make some lawyer rich. Mr. Goodrich (the lawyer) said I could beat it, probably, but it would cost me about $3,000. Goddamn!

Therapist/consultant: Hmm. And what's the problem as you see it, Maureen?

Maureen: The whole thing. How could he be so stupid as to get caught peeing in public? I guess that's what I'm angry about. I mean, we don't have a lot of money. I work at _____, you know? We've got a baby coming. How are we going to pay for all of this?

Therapist/consultant: Okay, the problem as you to see it now, is that Steven did something and it is going to cost a whole lot of money.

Steven: Yeah. And Mr. Goodrich said it was a good idea if I got some kind of alcohol counseling, you know, so that I could tell the judge I've been a good boy (laughter).

Therapist/consultant: Hmmm.

Maureen: It's going to cost us a fortune.

Therapist/consultant: Yeah, it sure is. But you know, this might not be the only problem. I mean . . .

Steven: I know what you're going to say. Quit drinking. Quit drinking!

Therapist/consultant: You've heard that before?

Steven: From my mother. She drives me to drink. Fuckin' right.

Therapist/consultant: Hmm. How so?

Steven: She's a jerk. A goddamn jerk.

Therapist/consultant: Hold on, remember our ground rule about name-calling. What do you think about that, Maureen? I mean, about Steve's mom?

Maureen: Not much. Steven likes to drink. I like to drink. He got caught peeing in public. Now we have to go through all of this bullshit and its embarrassing.

Therapist/consultant: Yeah, I bet it is. Well, who knows . . . (long pause). I guess your immediate problem is the legal charges. I can't say about anything else. At least for certain. I suspect something else.

Steven (with hostility): What else?

Therapist/consultant: Well, you might have a drinking problem. You might have some other, bigger problems. Could be anything. Family problems, physical problems, who knows . . . ?

Maureen: Yeah. Kidney problems (laughing). You really think (long pause) I'm an alcoholic? My granddaddy died of liver failure. So maybe I got it from him.

Therapist/consultant: I think we should keep an open mind. Maybe we need to find out some more information. Maybe then we'll have a clearer idea.

Steven: Maybe.

In this case the therapist/consultant was extraordinarily careful to avoid offering an interpretation that the family would summarily reject and could use as an excuse for treatment termination. He was also cautious to avoid advancing a single formation of the problem that might prove wrong in the future (e. g., "You're an alcoholic in denial"). When therapist/consultants advance a single explanation for the crisis at hand they often force themselves and the client family into a *premature problem foreclosure*. In effect they are saying to the family, "You are wrong and I am right, regardless of what we will find out in the future." Premature foreclosure of problem formation binds a family to an earlier mode of relating and explanation that may not reflect the changes that subsequent therapy will produce or potential causes that subsequent inquiry may uncover. It is especially problematic with the potentially resistant family.

A number of phrases are useful for offering the family a general explanation of their condition, yet avoiding a definitive commitment to causation. These include "As I see it now . . . ," or "Based upon what we're saying at this time . . . ." Often, it is helpful to explain to the family that diagnostic formulations can change during the course of treatment. To families in crisis, the therapist/consultants should appear competent and expert, though not omnipotent. Like Socrates with the slave boy of Meno, we need to convince the family that they have the answers; they just don't know that they do.

The importance of avoiding a premature foreclosure of problem formation is evident in the case study of the McCutcheon family, presented below. It was one of our numerous family therapy failures with resistant families.

Family Study 7.2. The McCutcheons

> Mr. Dwight McCutcheon, 39, a Midwestern factory worker, was evaluated in an emergency room by a crisis therapist. Mr. McCutcheon had just discontinued a four-day drinking bout and stated that he needed help for his substance usage. His nuclear family, Mrs. McCutcheon, age 36, Loretta, 17, and Scott, 15, were all involved in the interview. Each agreed that they were extremely worried regarding Mr. McCutcheon's drinking, and that they would do anything necessary to encourage his abstinence. Desperately concerned that the family would not follow through with treatment, the emergency worker continually claimed that the family could "return completely to normal" if Mr. McCutcheon would only begin Twelve-Step affiliation.

> Mr. McCutcheon began attending AA as well as weekly family therapy with a regular family therapist (other than their original emergency worker). The family became very involved

in recovery activities including Al Anon and Alateen. However, their present therapist noticed that no one in the family directly communicated to other family members regarding their feelings. The typical family pattern was to either be "passive aggressive" or to allow tension to build up until feelings exploded. In fact, the family would go out of its way to avoid spending idle time together when they might have to converse. Once involved in mutual activities, there was an extreme level of family tension.

Attempts to highlight these issues were unsuccessful. The family reiterated that only their first therapist, the crisis worker, was capable of understanding the real cause of their communication problems. "He told us it was the drinking and he saw right." The family terminated treatment at Mr. McCutcheon's 90th day of sobriety. Mr. McCutcheon stated flatly that the "record showed" that the "only family problem we got is the family disease of alcoholism. Period."

The next year was less kind to the family. Mrs. McCutcheon left her husband. Expressing herself in self-help clichés, she stated that she was "sick and tired of his stinking thinking." She had difficulty being more specific. Scott was later suspended from school for punching a classmate. He later apologized, but stated to his school counselor that he was "pissed off about things at home." Loretta was urged by friends at Alateen to seek individual therapy for her depression. Mr. McCutcheon had a major "slip" but still attends AA nightly.

Had the first therapist worker been less dogmatic regarding alcohol as the only family problem, the family's treatment outcome might have been different. Perhaps the family's progress might have also been fostered if their second therapist, the family therapist with whom they terminated, was better able to speak and understand the language of self-help modalities. Regardless, it is important for therapists to keep formulations tentative, so that family change is not stifled by adherence to target problems whose solutions are less important for present family functioning. As an aside, this case illustrates the frequent friction that family therapists have with self-help groups. It is important that family therapists be comfortable and familiar with the variety of available self-help modalities.

DECISION AVOIDANCE:
THE PRINCIPAL OBSTACLE
TO FAMILY PROBLEM SOLVING

A rather extensive literature has developed regarding family decision making. For our purposes, it is enough to state that families under stress will have difficulty making decisions, regardless of the degree of familial health or pathology. This factor is often overlooked by family therapists, who may interpret each incident of family avoidance of decision making as a diagnostic sign of a deeper problem. However, heightened stress can precipitate perseveration on tasks that people feel confident they can effectively perform, and avoidance of tasks with less perceived chance of success (McCown & Johnson, 1989). A common problem of families in crisis, especially resistant families, is the belief that they can decide not to decide. Therefore, many families in crisis will require firm support in order to make critical decisions.

The decision to *not* make a decision constitutes one component of a dysfunctional style of coping. Unfortunately, it is also a decision that may be highly rewarding. An example of this general principle is illustrated in Family Study 7.3, presented below. This case involves a 74-year-old patient with a gangrenous limb causing potentially fatal metabolic deterioration. The family is obviously stressed–perhaps overcome–by the enormity of the situation. They are called upon to make a decision whether to allow the patient to die or to try one last heroic effort to amputate his leg. However, they are having an extreme difficulty making this determination and seek any means available to delay making it.

Family Study 7.3. The Robertson Family

Mr. Robertson is a 74-year-old retired roofer who lives with his wife, Mrs. Helen Robertson, 71. Mr. Robertson has been hospitalized for three months with progressive gangrene related to a lengthy history of diabetes. Four surgeries have failed to halt the progress of the gangrene, and Mr. Robertson's condition continues to deteriorate. For at least one month, his mental status has been so poor that he is unable to make decisions for himself. Presently, he is in a semi-conscious state.

It is obvious to the entire family that Mr. Robertson has been suffering protractedly during his hospitalization. Some of the family members, as well as the medical personnel involved, have suggested that nature simply be allowed to take its course and that no more highly invasive procedures be done to save Mr. Robertson. This suggestion has generated an extreme conflict within the family between members who want Mr. Robertson "to die with peace and dignity" and those who "want to make sure Dad has a fighting chance."

The family's situation is complicated by the absence of a key family member, Heather, herself a physician on the opposite coast. Heather has been informally case-managing her father's care through frequent contacts with the physicians, family, and nursing staff. Heather's family describes her as "fiery and opinionated." Some of the medical staff have referred to her as "meddlesome and litigious." Mr. Robertson's initial physician quit the case in a dispute with Heather, acrimoniously adding to the family tension. In the opinion of the family's present physician, the family's inability to make timely decisions regarding Mr. Robertson's treatment has significantly contributed to his rapidly failing health.

The family has been joined by a social worker who has been consulting with them regarding their father's medical management. A family meeting has been called by the social worker involving the entire available family and the patient's primary care physician, Dr. Thomlinson, who herself is ambivalent about the prospects for surgery on Mr. Robertson. Heather, who has promised to be available for the family meeting, remains absent and has not answered several telephone calls.

Therapist/consultant: As you know, Mr. Robertson's internist said that we have to make a decision about his leg. Dr. Thomlinson thinks we need to make the decision now.

Dr. Thomlinson: Yes, as I have told some of you, there is some disagreement about whether we should proceed with further surgery. Basically, this is the way I see it. If we do have Dr. Tenansky operate, the chances are maybe, well, I wouldn't say they are good. But they are at least chances. On the other hand, if we do operate, we may simply prolong Mr. Robertson's suffering a few more days or weeks. To this date, surgery hasn't done well. I think maybe we need to make a decision.

Therapist/consultant: What do you think, Mrs. Robertson?

Mrs. R.: (long hesitation) I want to leave it to the doctors. They know best.

Rob R.: (son, age 31). I'm for leaving it with the doctors.

Therapist/consultant: Well, their concern is that they don't know your father. They don't know how he would adjust to this severe of an amputation on his other leg at his age. And then there is the issue of whether we would prolong his suffering.

Mrs. R.: Maybe we can call in another doctor for some more advice.

Therapist/consultant: That's a good idea, although I'm afraid that after reading the medical history they'd decide the same thing.

Dr. Thomlinson: From a medical perspective, if we are going to operate we need to do it soon. The sooner we remove the gangrene, the more likelihood that Mr. Robertson will recover.

Mrs. R.: Let's wait for Heather to arrive.

Therapist/consultant: How do you two feel about that?

John: Heather won't get here until tomorrow. Mom, the doctor said we got to decide now.

Rob R.: I don't think we can make this kind of decision without Heather.

Therapist/consultant: Why?

Rob R.: What if we are wrong? What if we do something and it doesn't work out? I think the family needs to be together on this one.

Therapist/consultant: Can you just call her? On the phone.

Rob R.: I think she needs to be here, you know, to get a feel for what is happening.

Therapist/consultant: I think we need to remember what Dr. Thomlinson said. Not deciding to do something is basically making a choice. Is that right?

Dr. Thomlinson: Pretty much so, yeah. Um . . . We have a limited window of opportunity, as it were, to work. The sooner we operate, if that's what we decide to do, the better his chances.

Therapist/consultant: Can you give us some better indication of what the chances are? I mean, maybe in percentages. So it can help us make a decision . . .

Dr. Thomlinson: Well, I'm not really . . . I mean, such things are inexact–but . . .

Therapist/consultant: It would be very helpful to the family if you could–give us some indication . . .

Dr. Thomlinson: Again, we don't want to put firm numbers . . . But I would say maybe that if we don't operate we are talking about maybe a one in twenty chance of leaving the hospital. Maybe less. With surgery, maybe 20%, maybe 25% percent. Again, those numbers are just estimates . . . might be way off.

Therapist/consultant: So essentially, you feel we are doubling Mr. Robertson's chances for survival by operating?

Dr. Thomlinson: At least. On the other hand, if we simply prolong his agony, we're not doing much good. Unquestionably, he will live longer if we operate. The real issue is whether he will live well enough to warrant the surgery. And if he does live, can he adjust to life without a limb?

Therapist/consultant: It seems that we need to make a decision today. What do you all think?

The Robertsons demonstrate the familiar pattern of people who are in crisis who do not want to make a decision. However, in about

30 percent of cases, resistant families will demonstrate an opposite tendency, that of premature decision making. These families may come to the first or subsequent sessions with an agenda, and as we have indicated earlier, if the agenda is not met, abruptly terminate services. Or, they may seize the first solution offered to them and become inflexible regarding the possibility of examining other alternatives. The goal of the therapist/consultant is to avoid both extremes and foster the family's informed decision making regarding problem resolution.

Optimal decision making involves the weighing of alternatives and obtaining feedback regarding their desirability. Resistant families are usually lacking competency in these areas. The anxiety or impulsivity of these families may be so high that it is difficult for them to delay making a decision. Additionally, poor family communications, mistrust, problems with roles, and general family tension may make individual members less receptive to feedback by those within and outside of the family. As a result the resistant family is often characterized by three attributes: (1) individual decisions are made quickly, without regard to adequate consideration of alternatives; (2) there is little feedback or discussion among family members regarding possibilities for other actions; consequently, (3) there is apt to be little family consensus regarding which decisions are appropriate. Indeed, another reason that resistant families may prematurely terminate from treatment lies in the lack of initial consensus regarding need for treatment.

PROBLEM-FOCUSED COPING: THE FAMILY GENERATES ITS OWN ANSWERS

Coping refers to cognitive and behavioral ways in which people attempt to manage stressors (Lazarus & Folkman, 1984). Many researchers designate at least two different types of coping. Problem-focused coping seeks to improve the crisis situation by providing alternative behaviors (Nezu, Nezu, & Perri, 1989). Emotion-focused coping seeks to manage the emotional distress associated with crises (Lazarus & Folkman, 1984). The decision-making phase for people in crisis can include a modicum of forced coping where individuals are assisted in generating a number of potential coping variables and choosing between them. These can either be problem-focused solutions or emotion-focused solutions.

The essence of our intervention with resistant families is to ask them to generate their own problem-focused solutions to their situations. Often, when resistant families are told that this will be their task, they are dumbfounded! They will appear stymied and baffled, and may even become hostile. After all, aren't therapists supposed to have all of the answers? Indeed, as one of our clients recently said, "Why the hell else do I employ you, except to think for me?"

Through the process of problem-*focused* coping we communicate that the family is expected to generate one or more potential solutions to their own problems. The therapist/consultant firmly, but gently, directs the family to potential behaviors that may solve their problems and then helps them decide which are appropriate. In this process the therapist/consultant is there to assist the family, but not to make decisions for them. The onus of choosing and following a particular course of action is gradually directed from the therapist toward the family. As the family gains confidence in themselves and their ability to problem solve, they will be more likely to draw upon their own resources, as opposed to relying on professional help to assist them in coping with problems of family processes. Furthermore, as families gain experience in successful coping they are less likely to resort to dysfunctional mechanisms which, as we have argued, ultimately cause resistance.

The notion that we expect the family to solve its own difficulties is rarely initially accepted by families who are in a crisis. This is especially true for the resistant system, which is quite comfortable with having others make plans for it, only to thwart the plans at a later date. Therefore, it is important this expectation is communicated with utmost sensitivity and sense of routineness and normalcy. The therapist/consultant should make it clear that the family, and not the professional, will provide solutions. After formulating the problem, the therapist/consultant can use a phrase such as "Now that we all know what the problem is, we need us, and especially you, to solve it." The role of the therapist/consultant is to coach and clarify, not to dictate future behavior. A strategic use of phrasing can communicate this sentiment subtly yet definitively.

Only when a family *cannot* generate its own potential coping strategies should the therapist/consultant directly intervene and suggest options. In one study of resistant families (in progress)* we found that less than 10% of families are completely unable to generate any of their own potential solutions to problems. In other words, nine out of ten families can generate at least one viable solution to their problems during a crisis situation. The therapist/consultant may have to reiterate his or her expectation several times to obtain this degree of compliance. However, the sensitive, yet persistent, clinician can usually succeed with perseverance.

In about 10 percent of cases (at least in the four treatment settings we have studied in detail) families will not be able to generate even one solution to their problems. Clinical experience suggests this is most likely to occur when the therapist/consultant has not sufficiently defused the crisis, or has erred by allowing the most powerful family member or members to dominate the crisis session to the exclusion of others. If this is the case, it may be necessary to spend additional time interviewing family members or asking them to formulate their view of the family's problems. This will usually generate a number of suggestions regarding the family's problems which can then be rephrased to appropriately reflect potential solutions.

A more pervasive problem than the family with no solutions is the system that generates only one or two poor choices. For example, a therapist/consultant may not be able to help a resistant family move beyond the problem-focused choice of reducing family strains by "putting our crazy son away forever," or "sending Mom to a nursing home once and for all." Resistant families sometimes have emotional and behavioral "tunnel vision" in the sense they may seize upon one solution to their crisis and are inflexible in generating additional options. Furthermore, families will sometimes display tunnel vision if they are dominated by a single powerful member. The antidote to this lies in increasing the quantity and quality of family involvement.

An advantage of including many family members in the crisis session is that the variety of opinions usually facilitates a larger number of

---

*Data obtained from a study in progress.

potential coping responses. In our work with individuals and families, we have found that each additional family member contributes approximately two unique potential solutions. This includes children above eight, who sometimes are the best sources for problem-focused solutions. Obviously, the more family members present, the more likely a viable solution to the family's problems will be considered and eventually endorsed by the family system. It is also helpful to begin the discussion of decision alternatives by first soliciting the input from the least powerful person in the family system, thereby dissuading psychological or emotional blocks that might follow the pronouncement of the most powerful family member.

The most common problem regarding family problem solving is that they will generate several irrelevant ideas regarding optimal methods for coping with stressors. For example, one recent family we worked with that was faced with an intractable 13-year-old daughter suggested the following possible solutions: (1) hospitalization (2) psychotropic medication administration (3) jail (4) a lobotomy, and (5) emancipation from the home. Obviously, none of these were particularly helpful, and the skilled therapist needs to further prod the family until at least one potentially useful solution is generated by a family member. In this case, the therapist/consultant had to send the family home overnight to come up with additional solutions. The family eventually recalled a once recommended behavioral management system for their daughter and the therapist/consultant assisted the family with implementation of this idea.

It may also be necessary for the resistant family to be restrained regarding premature decision making. A useful technique to avoid is to have each family member generate only one or two potential coping solutions. This is most useful for the extraverted or impulsive family that seems unable to focus. Sometimes this should be done in writing and individually, so that family members avoid the tendency to acquiesce to the most powerful person in the family system. These potential solutions can be discussed in a family framework, with the most viable ones being chosen as courses of action.

A major concern is management irrelevant or harmful solutions the family produces without discouraging families from continuing to search for answers on their own. The therapist/consultant will certainly hear a number of superfluous, and seemingly inconsequential ideas generated by the family during this phase of the crisis session. If this occurs, he or she should politely attempt to allow other family members to challenge the appropriateness or relevance of the proffered option. In extreme cases where family members lack the expertise, cognitive sophistication, or ability to do so, the therapist/consultant should tactfully intervene and assume a more active role in solution generation. Although we will shortly wish to foster discussion regarding the feasibility of alternatives, this discussion should be restrained until after a number of alternatives have been generated. What we strive to avoid is the situation where one or two potential coping strategies are being presented and then immediately torpedoed by other family members as silly, unworkable, or crazy. It is important to keep as many ideas "on the table" as possible, which serves to avoid power struggles between family members or between the family and the therapist/consultant.

As discussed above, resistant families in crisis generally cannot generate any solutions at all. This most frustrating situation will occur in about 10 percent of all crisis cases. After a period of time the therapist/consultant can legitimately suggest a number of potential solutions and request input and decision regarding their viability. Such families may need to be prompted a few times, but usually can succeed in generating their own potential options following some prompting and modeling of the concept by the therapist.

In the Family Study below, the Robertsons (continued), the therapist/consultant skillfully employs problem-focused coping to make the family choose a solution to their present crisis. Many of the techniques discussed above are employed in this interchange.

Family Study 7.3. The Robertsons (continued)

Therapist/consultant: It seems like we all need to come up with some sort of solution to the surgery problem. Frankly, it has to be your decision, since you are the family. But I'll help as best as I can.

Mrs. R.: I just wish we could ask Dr. Thomlinson to wait a few days.

John R.: At least until we can talk to Heather.

Therapist/consultant: Hmmm. I'm not certain that's a good idea or not. Remember, not deciding is the same as deciding. This might be what we want to do. It might not be. Let's see if we can think of what our options . . . all our options are.

Rob R.: We could go ahead with the surgery. Or we could call in another expert.

John R.: Maybe we would be better if we called Heather and talked with her.

Therapist/consultant: Hmm. Anything else? Other ideas?

Mrs. R.: We could get another opinion. From another doctor. I don't like the one we have now.

Therapist/consultant: Okay. We have several choices. Do nothing. Call Heather. Get more opinion. Go with the surgery. Any thoughts?

Mrs. R.: I say we call Heather.

John. R.: I agree.

Therapist/consultant: Do we have her number?

Mrs. R.: Yes, I have it somewhere, her work number.

Note that the therapist/consultant wisely prepares the family for the possibility that this initial coping choice will not work. He mentally rehearses with the family the possibility that Heather may not be available. This is an extremely important step to undertake when the therapist/consultant believes, even remotely, that the family's first coping response may not prove viable. In this manner, the therapist/consultant is helping the family to prepare for the fact their preferred means of coping may not be tenable. This is simply another method of enhancing the controllability of the stress involved.

Therapist/consultant: Before we call Heather, I want to ask, what will we do when, well, if we can't get hold of her. I remember speaking with her yesterday and she said something about not being around today.

Mrs. R.: You mean, if we can't get her on the telephone?

Therapist/consultant: Yes. What will we do next?

John R.: Well, let's wait 'til that happens before we decide.

Therapist/consultant: I think we might need to consider it before we try. That way if we don't get her, we can still decide what to do.

John R.: I think if we do not get her, we need to wait a while, maybe try later.

Rob R.: No, that's the same as not deciding. Isn't that right Dr. Thomlinson?

Dr. Thomlinson: I think the decision has to belong to the family. But yes, if you wait a long time, you've already decided. That's the point I've been trying to make. If you wait, even another day or so, there is much less chance the surgery will work and much greater chance that the patient will not benefit from it. I would be more comfortable if we decided today.

Rob R.: Now?

Dr. Thomlinson: Within a few hours.

Therapist/consultant: I suggest that we all decide that if we cannot locate Heather, we make a decision in the next few hours. Dr. Thomlinson? When do they need to know about our decision regarding operation?

Dr. Thomlinson: I suppose as soon as possible. They would have to schedule the O.R. Even for an emergency, it's important to schedule it. Anesthesiology would have to be called and the like.

John R.: Why? I mean it is an emergency.

Dr. Thomlinson: The longer the surgeon and the anesthesiologist have to prepare—the better things can be. The anesthesiologist, for example, he needs to review the records and so on. This is not routine surgery. Mr. Robertson is in pretty poor physical condition. There are numerous risks. Let me stress that again. There are risks.

Therapist/consultant: So it sounds like if we can't get hold of Heather, we need to make a decision within a hour or so.

Dr. Thomlinson: Yes, I think that would be best.

Rob R.: Okay, before we call Heather, do we all agree that if we can't get hold of her, we will decide to make a decision by, let's give it maybe 'til 3:00. Okay?

Mrs. R.: Yeah. Okay.

Rob R.: We have to decide something.

John R.: But Heather said to wait 'til she gets here.

Therapist/consultant: It's your decision. But if we wait much longer, we will have no decision. None to make.

At this point in the interview a number of potential options may be "floating around" among family members. The next goal of the therapist/consultant is to reduce these options so that they can be incorporated into a manageable contract for the family. We call this process *problem-solving closure*. The aim of problem-solving closure is to leave the family with a formulated behavioral plan for solving mutually agreed upon goals. This closure should result in plan that reflects, as much as possible, the family's own attempts to solve its problems. Usually, this plan should be made in writing. When it is, we call it the *Family Behavioral Contract* and it always involves a specific course of action for family members to follow during the crisis period. Chapter Eight will discuss the Family Behavioral Contract at greater length.

To the novice family therapist/consultant it may seem difficult to obtain consensus or closure from family members regarding which potential action choices they should pursue. Interestingly, this decision is usually not as difficult for families to make as it first appears. Even very conflictual and high risk families can typically agree to attempt a unified set of behaviors, at least for a specified period of time. Obviously, the skilled therapist/consultant gently guides the family's decision making regarding which options are appropriate and most likely help the family meet its needs.

The therapist/consultant can use a number of techniques to subtly reinforce one potential course of action over another and thereby obtain closure. Nonverbal techniques are often effective. For example, the therapist/consultant can nod especially forcefully or otherwise show enthusiasm when a particularly promising potential family behavior is expressed. The therapist/consultant can also express direct verbal approval, such as exclaiming "Now, that's a good idea!" when the family attempts to decide on a particular behavior. More introverted families generally benefit from a lower keyed verbalization, such as "Hmm, that really might work," or "Now, that's an interesting idea."

The therapist/consultant can also provide feedback regarding each potential behavior. Usually this advice should be indirect. For example, it is best to request the family to point out *why* a particular idea is unworkable rather than explain or otherwise inform the family directly. When advice is given during this stage of the interview it should always be presented in a normalized and considerate fashion.

If the resistant family cannot reach consensus, it may be helpful to simply have them vote on what they will do next. Voting is most helpful where there are a number of equally powerful adult family members who disagree among themselves. This usually occurs when the extended family is assembled during a crisis. Voting is less appropriate when the family is composed mostly of adolescents and children and a potential goal of therapy is to strengthen generational boundaries and power.

The least desirable technique is for the therapist/consultant to choose which potential behavioral suggestions the family should pursue. However, this is occasionally unavoidable, especially for very conflictual or cognitively unsophisticated families. However, whenever possible, the family should be afforded at least the illusion of control regarding their choices. One strategic way to accomplish this is to narrow the family's choice of options down to three or four, all but one of which are unsatisfactory, absurd, or otherwise nonreinforcing to the family. Here, the therapist/consultant can take liberties to invent any potential behavior he or she can think of, as long as it is not likely to be endorsed by the family. This is illustrated in the Family Study of the Robertson family, below.

Family Study 7.3. The Robertsons (continued)

Mrs. R.: I just can't make a decision. About this. What if he dies . . . . I just can't. I mean, I just don't know. I want to wait until Heather arrives. It won't be long.

Therapist/consultant: Well, I guess we could decide to get some closure here. Or we can simply let Mr. Robertson die. Maybe that's the best course of action. Yeah, that way, we solve a lot of problems.

John R.: I don't understand. What are you . . .

Therapist/consultant: Simple. No one makes a decision. So we just all agree to let Dad die. I propose we vote on it. Do we let him die, or do we decide to take additional action?

Mrs. R.: Oh, you're just horrible, talking like that! I can't stand it.

Therapist/consultant: Then in that case, let me cast your vote for letting your husband die. Okay, we have two choices, surgery, or death. I vote for death. Now, I'm not the family, but to me it's pretty clear. Let him die. What about the family?

Mrs. Robertson: No, no, no! I say we go with the surgery.

Therapist/consultant: I guess we disagree. Well, let's vote on it.

The family voted in "secret ballot" and decided on surgery.

EGO-LENDING:
MAKING DECISIONS FOR THE FAMILY

As we have indicated, some families are so dysfunction they have extreme difficulty even with the task of generating potential options to solve their problems. In some settings, it is common to observe families that have difficulties meeting even their most instrumental needs, such as food and shelter. For severely impaired families or families in extreme crisis, the therapist/consultant may need to act forcefully and invasively, essentially "lending" his or her ego to the client family to make decisions for them. In ego-lending, the therapist/consultant makes important decisions for the family with the realization that this process is potentially counter-productive, since it disempowers the family. On the other hand, the chaotic dysfunctionality that accompanies many resistant families, or that ensues from a catastrophic instrumental stressor, may require the therapist/consultant to temporarily sacrifice empowerment for the more immediate goal of problem solving.

When families in instrumental crisis cannot adequately make decisions, the therapist/consultant *must* do this for them. This is most likely to occur when a family encounters extraordinary and unexpected instrumental stressors, such as a sudden death or a natural disaster. On the other hand, ego lending is almost never appropriate for perceptual emergencies, except with the most dys-functional systems. Even then, it should be undertaken with ex-treme care since the goal to allow the family to solve their own problems still remains.

Ego-lending may also be necessary when an important and pow-erful member of the family system is absent from the crisis session. Because the family respects, defers to, and even fears this member, they may be unable to make provisions for even basic survival in the absence of this member. For example, women who have been abused by their spouse may be afraid to make elementary family decisions in the absence of the abusing partner. We have been told of several accounts where crisis workers intervening following the San Francisco earthquake of 1989 found that such women would not consent to emergency medical treatment for themselves or their children without consulting their husbands! Many therapists who work in women's shelters routinely note a similar phenomenon. In these cases, the therapist/consultant has no magic solution to guar-antee that he or she is acting in the family's best interests. He or she simply must weigh the family's instrumental needs and, if deemed appropriate, decide what to do for the family. Under these circum-stances, it is usually best to be subtle with the family members.

Ego-lending, in essence, represents a therapeutic retreat. The crisis worker realizes that he or she needs to retrench and resume the role of supportive therapist rather than continue the engagement towards systems consultant. Despite this, ego-lending may sometimes involve forcing a family to make a decision. This too, must be tactfully done. The Robertson case illustrates the desirability of this subtlety.

Family Study 7.3. The Robertsons (continued)

The therapist/consultant contacted all of the appropriate physicians involved and told them that the family decided on surgery for Mr. Robertson. However, during this time, Heather's nurse left a message instructing the family not to make any determination until they talked with her in person on the following day. The message further indicated that Heather intended to fly out this evening, but that she would be unavailable until she arrived at the hospital the following morning.

This message made the family reconsider their decision to operate. They then colluded to return to their earlier plan of waiting a few more hours before deciding anything. Mrs. Robertson informed the surgeon's answering service of this new development. Upon hearing this new development, the surgeon on the case, Dr. Tenansky, became extremely angry and stated he would refuse to operate if contacted past the previously agreed upon deadline. He then called back a few minutes later, stating he was contacting the hospital attorney to obtain a court order for surgery on Mr. Robertson.

The therapist/consultant knew that if he shared this information with the family, this would simply increase their confusion and their resolve to do nothing. Instead, he gently reminded them of their previous deadline regarding their decision to be made–with or without Heather's input.

He then asked the family to go off alone together and decide for themselves what needed to be done for Mr. Robertson. On their own, the family contacted the surgeon about the possibility of delaying this decision. Dr. Tenansky reiterated to the family that in his opinion, Mr. Robertson needed surgery and that the family needed to give immediate consent.

The family eventually decided to vote again on the surgery, and asked the therapist/consultant to moderate the voting. On the "initial ballot," all three members abstained. The therapist/consultant again reminded them that by not deciding, they were in reality making an irrevocable decision. He directly intervened into the family's decision-making process by telling them that they were "not allowed to decide not to decide." A second ballot was conducted, this time with no abstentions allowed. All three family members voted for surgery.

Heather arrived the next day and was livid that the decision to operate was made in her absence. However, the family stood stalwart and reminded her of the time constraints. Eventually, Mr. Robertson was discharged home and made a moderately satisfactory adjustment.

In the therapist/consultant's view, it was most important that the family present a unified front to both the physicians involved in the case and to Heather. The therapist/consultant realized that responsibility for much of the daily care of Mr. Robertson would ultimately reside within the immediate family. Therefore, they needed to be reasonably comfortable and satisfied with their decision. However, because the family was so reticent to make a decision, they needed a degree of limit setting that they apparently could not provide for themselves. The therapist, in a moderate act of ego lending, performed this task for them.

Novice therapists frequently become involved in making too many decisions for the family in crisis. In the case of perceptual crises, the resistant family invariably uses this overinvolvement as an excuse to terminate subsequent treatment. We do not advocate ego lending unless there is a substantial instrumental danger to the family system or an individual member. Instead, it is more useful for families in an instrumental crisis who are on the brink of making poor decisions to be encouraged to use a "cooling off period" of a few hours or days. The therapist/consultant should recontact the family after they have had time to consider impending actions and before they have acted in an irrevocable manner. There are few exceptions to this, and typically involve cases where the family can irrevocably harm someone who is not capable of giving informed consent. These situations will be discussed later.

WHEN THE FAMILY DECIDES POORLY:
THE CONSULTANT STANCE

One of the most common events in family crisis therapy occurs when the therapist and family do not agree on an optimal course of action. Despite the therapist/consultant's best efforts and even ego lending, the family insists on making a decision that, in the therapist/consultant's opinion is less than optimal or appropriate. Examples are numerous to any practicing family clinician: the family that insists on discontinuing their schizophrenic adolescent son's medication, the battered woman that won't press charges against her husband, and the family of a substance abuser who continues to enable their abusing member. Furthermore, additional problem solving often seems only to reiterate the family's desire to follow their chosen course of resistance.

When situations such as these occur, several therapeutic options exist. Some therapist/consultants attempt to employ the illusion of choice regarding crisis alternatives. This might occur when an alcoholic is given the "choice" of either attending AA or undergoing involuntary commitment. Sometimes this technique works, at least briefly, and may be worth a try.

Other crisis therapists directly suggest alternative strategies to the family and maintain an open door to them until their preferred problem-focused solution fails. Subsequent crisis sessions are used to try new options, until the family endorses a course of action that will truly help solve their present and distal problems. Unfortunately, this general procedure often fails with treatment resistant families who simply may drop out of crisis intervention just as they do with longer-term therapy.

Still other therapists increase ego lending, augmenting their involvement with the family so that the system will not fail. Sometimes this approach is necessary. As we stated previously, families experiencing traumatic instrumental crises cannot be allowed to continue dysfunctional behavior. This is especially true for cases of incest, child or elder abuse, or where someone in the family system is brain compromised and cannot make an informed consent. When this technique succeeds, the family may have overcome a present problem, but will have learned very little from the crisis other than that they are helpless and need professional support. If the family is crisis-prone, they will invariably "recycle" with yet another problem.

From our perspective the most useful response to the fact that resistant families make poor decisions is simply to shift gears completely and act as a consultant to the family system. Even in instances where the family is making a mistake that may ultimately prove harmful, the crisis therapist/consultant needs to emotionally disinvest him or herself and assume the role of family advisor. At this point the "consultant's" job is to advise the family of the reasonableness of their choice and the likelihood that it will meet their needs.

The abrupt shift into the role of family consultant is illustrated below, in Family Study 7.4.

Family Study 7.4. The Whitmans

> Carole and John Whitman, 29 and 33, were both habitual alcohol abusers. On weekends, they would get drunk and fight, sometimes quite seriously. Then, in an all-too-familiar pattern, they would tearfully reunite and vow never to fight again. Sometimes the police were involved. Occasionally, the fights involved a trip to the emergency room.
>
> During one of these sessions, the emergency room physician suggested that they be seen by the on-call social worker, a crisis therapist. The therapist evaluated the couple (which by now had made up) and suggested that they spend a few hours apart, at least until they sobered up. The couple was highly resistent to this suggestion. However, the therapist handled this resistance adroitly and diplomatically, and was eventually able to convince the couple of the probability that they would hit each other again. The transcript below illustrates some of the interchange.
>
> *Carole:* No fucking way. I want to go home. I want to go home. I'm going home, goddamn it.
>
> *Therapist/consultant:* Carole, you said you'd listen to what I had to say, remember? John, remember that?

John: Come on, hurry up. You said we could go home.

Therapist/consultant: And you promised me that you would go to your mother's house, at least until you sobered up.

John: Okay, okay, I changed my mind. I am sober, anyway. Want me to walk a white line? (laughs).

Therapist/consultant: John, you can do what you want to do. The police have decided not to press charges, not this time. But you need to remember, you guys told me you've punched each other maybe ten times this past year. Ten times. And each time you've been drunk.

Carole: Yeah, I know . . . but we're not drinking now.

Therapist/consultant: But your blood alcohol level is well over the legal limit–something like–let me look at the number–.22. You are two and a half times the legal limit for being drunk.

Carole: So?

Therapist/consultant: So when you've been like this before, there's been problems. You're like this now. So there might be problems.

Carole: Hey. I can handle it. I'm a big girl (laughs). I take care of my own . . .

Therapist/consultant: I know you are. And I can't make the decision for you. But look. I'm an expert. That's why I work here. And I know that when you drink, sometimes you beat up on each other. If you want to risk it, I can't stop you, as long as you don't drive home. But the sensible thing to do is to take the day off from each other. Get away. Make up tomorrow, when you're sober. It's not safe otherwise.

John: Hmmm. I could go stay with my mother.

Therapist/consultant: Maybe both of you should go stay somewhere. Bruises take a long time to heal.

Carole: I keep telling you, I'm not drunk. Just fuck off! I mean it! I'm going home.

Therapist/consultant: Your blood test says you are, and that's what I go by.

John: Maybe she's right.

Carole: I just want to go to sleep.

Therapist/consultant: Then do it here. We'll get you admitted if you choose, or, we can see, maybe she could sleep it off at the (Women's) Shelter.

John: What if I don't want her to? You going to stop us if we leave?

Therapist/consultant: No. It's your lives, not mine. I won't keep you from making your own mistakes, if you choose to.

John: You mean you won't get us arrested or anything?

Therapist/consultant: Like I said, it's your decision. But I think I need to remind you of the past. Legally, the doctor may want to keep her until her alcohol drops below .10. I'll check. But after that, it's up to you. But it's not a good idea.

Carole: Oh, just let me go to sleep, okay? Maybe he's right. Go on home, John. I'll see you in the morning.

The above Family Study had a fortuitous ending. It should not be used to obscure the fact that families under stress–especially resistant families– will make mistakes. As *consultants* to families our philosophy regarding our responsibility to them has evolved from that advocated by traditional family therapists. *Unless the family is faced with a serious instrumental crisis we no longer believe we should assume responsibility for families making mistakes.* In other words, unless there is the imminent likelihood that someone will get hurt, we no longer try to rescue families from their bad choices.

This may seem to be an untraditional stance for family therapists. It certainly goes against the grain of crisis therapists who have practice in ego lending and may believe they must assume responsibility for the family in crisis. Unfortunately, making decisions the family will not adhere to is typically not helpful. Families must be allowed to make their own decisions, even if these decisions are "wrong," i.e., those the consultant or therapist would not choose.

The defining characteristic of our approach with resistant families is that we let them make their own mistakes, if they choose to do so. We no longer believe the therapist/consultant must or even can "save" or otherwise rescue the resistant family. Instead, the consultant's job is to provide the family with informed choices regarding their present and future behavior. When we consult with families we essentially employ our expertise to help them "reality test" whether their intended course of action will succeed in meeting their needs. We offer our expert opinion, and attempt to rationally convince the family that the opinion is valid. An example of this is presented in the Family Study below.

Family Study 7.5. The Thompson Family

Gary Thompson, 39, and his wife Fran, 43, both Midwestern factory workers, were concerned about the behavior of their sons, Gerald, 18, and Lonnie, 16. Gerald had quit his job as a video game mechanic to follow a particular rock group around the country. Although he had little savings, Gerald took off in his car, with the intention of seeing every one of the group's shows.

Lonnie had been smoking marijuana on a daily basis and was recently arrested for attempting to break into an adult bookstore video machine. When not on drugs, Lonnie spent most of his time in his room, sculpting or charcoal sketching.

The Thompson family sought an initial emergency evaluation following Lonnie's arrest. The therapist/consultant formulated that the family was marked by a number of potential structural problems. Furthermore, they had a history of dropping out of previous therapies. They were, in short, a high risk family. The therapist/consultant suggested to the family that they needed ongoing family work to solve their difficulties. Both parents continually balked at this option and instead demanded that the therapist/consultant "get Lonnie declared incorrigible."

"Let the little bastard stay in jail," Mr. Thompson stated.

At this point the therapist/consultant shifted roles to that of family consultant. He explained in a calm manner that Lonnie would be released regardless of what anyone did. He then reiterated each of the family's options, including no treatment for Lonnie, individual therapy and family therapy. He then stressed how the first two options had failed in the past and would likely fail again. Finally, he highlighted the fee schedule and attendance requirements that family therapy would involve. The family was still unconvinced.

The therapist/consultant then respectfully suggested to the family that further interviewing would serve no more use. He told the family flatly, that in all probability, their problems would get worse if the family was not involved in therapy. He then suggested that if they changed their minds, to give him a call at a later date. The family failed to follow up on any of these measures and continued to deteriorate.

The reader may be struck by the manner in which the crisis worker handled the Thompson family, compared with the generally supportive tone presented with earlier families. Charisma, empathy, sensitivity, and verve may be helpful for initially defusing crises, and to a lesser extent, in assessment and problem-solving. However, by the end of the problem-solving portion of the crisis interview a new set of therapeutic skills are required. When attempting to consult with families the following guidelines are useful.

First, we highlight the necessity of speaking in a neutral and unemotional tone of voice. Pressuring or attempting to persuade the family should be avoided. This is evident in the excellent technique of the therapist/consultant in Family Study 7.3. It is also often useful to speak in shorter, readily comprehensible sentences which emphasize facts, rather than feelings. Consultation is an intellectual exchange, rather than an emotional and empathetic one. When consulting with families the therapist is essentially advising them of the reasonableness of their plans, not trying to persuade them.

Secondly, our experience has suggested this inviolate rule: Do not promise anything that you cannot reasonably guarantee. It is usually best to speak in terms of probabilities. This is especially true for high risk families, since they may be seeing you again very soon regardless of what you do or say. There are few things in crisis intervention work more uncomfortable than to have family say to you "You told us that if we only did X, Y, & Z, our problems would be solved. We did these things. We still have the problem." How much better it is to have spoken in terms of probabilities! Phrases such as "most chance of," "a good possibility that," or "best choice" are much more realistic than shallow promises that the family will be cured by specific recommended actions.

Third, we also stress that a nonjudgmental attitude should be maintained throughout consultation. This may be extremely difficult to maintain when families make mistakes. However, we believe it is better to allow resistant families to err on their own rather than to disempower them.

Finally, and most importantly, the family should *accurately* be apprised of the likelihood of success generated by their chosen action. This appraisal should be based upon both the therapist/consultant's experience and the social science literature. The therapist/consultant should respond honestly when he or she does not know the answer. Honesty and realism are the best techniques for breaking down the resistance of family systems that do not want to change. This is illustrated in a continuation of the Family Study of the Thompsons.

Family Study 7.5. The Thompsons (continued)

Two crises later, it has become apparent that Mr. Thompson is a chronic gambler, spending large portions of his paycheck at the local dog track and making frequent "business trips" to Las Vegas. His attempts to control this behavior have proven ineffective. Recently, he has been threatening suicide as a solution to his mounting financial losses.

This session was prompted by concerns expressed by Mr. Thompson's friend, Vince, and priest, Father Jack O'Reilly, both of whom are in attendance. Fran, however, is not present, and has recently left Mr. Thompson for his erstwhile best friend, Jesse. Naturally, this has added to Mr. Thompson's depression and he has begun to drink heavily on a daily basis. He is slightly drunk during this session.

Both Father Jack and Vince have come up with the idea that Mr. Thompson needs to attend Gamblers Anonymous, an organization that Mr. Thompson has tried, but violently disliked. The atmosphere in the room is quite tense.

Mr. Thompson: Look, to me, it's all bullshit. Sorry, Father (laughs). Twelve-steps and all. You see, I was brought up on a farm. We were taught to be tough. Hard working. To me, you either do something or you don't. You don't mess around. And so when I think I need to quit, I'll quit.

Father Jack: It doesn't work that way. Your problem is bigger than you are.

Mr. Thompson: Oh, that's a load of bullcrap. I used to drink a case a night. And I quit, you see? No problem! And when I think playing the dogs is a problem, I'll quit. No problem!

Therapist/consultant: So you feel you have control over your gambling, just like you did over your drinking?

Mr. Thompson: You got it. C-O-N-T-R-O-L.

Vince: Gary, you didn't start gambling until after you quit drinking. You know, when we stopped hanging out at Denny's and the Log Cabin (local bars) and those places–I guess it is partly my fault. Gary and I used to be big boozers.

Therapist/consultant: So Vince, what you are saying is that Mr. Thompson's gambling and drinking are related.

Vince: Yeah, I guess so. Yeah. You could say.

Mr. Thompson: Bullshit. Hey, you want to try me out? I'll go for the rest of the year without gambling. I used to go to AA, and then I quit that stuff. And I can drink one or two beers with no problem. I mean it, too!

Therapist/consultant: Hmm. Okay, we have two suggestions. One is that Mr. Thompson needs to go to Gamblers Anonymous. The other is that he can quit on his own, like he evidently quit drinking on his own.

Mr. Thompson: Yeah.

Therapist/consultant: Well, to tell you the truth, in my experience, folks who seem to go from one addiction to another, like you seemed to have, have a much worse time of it. Frankly, they seem to be sicker, to have more problems.

Vince: What does that mean?

Therapist/consultant: I mean that people who go from abusing one thing to another, like Mr. Thompson seems to have done with alcohol and now with gambling, these people need professional treatment. And, I'll be honest, sometimes treatment doesn't work. Multiple addictions are much more serious. Period.

Vince: You think?

Father Jack: So you are saying that if Gary gets help now, he can be cured?

Therapist/consultant: To be honest, no. People with multiple addictions are rarely ever "cured." They learn to control their addictions. Almost always, this happens with a Twelve-Step program.

Mr. Thompson: And what if I don't go to AA? I hate that shit.

Vince: Or GA?

Therapist/consultant: We can't say for sure. But I think you probably won't make it.

Mr. Thompson: What do you mean, won't make it? I won't kill myself. I already promised that. If I had wanted to, I would have before, you know. (Angrily) Are you in AA? I don't know whether it's true or not, you hear this bullshit all the time from AA.

Therapist/consultant: I'm being objective about this. What you choose to do is your decision. I hope you do the right thing. But it's up to you.

Mr. Thompson: I mean you hear this shit from people in the program–sorry, Father. You hear this stuff–people tell you all this and you know, you hear it from people in the program. Like I've never heard from someone who wasn't an alcoholic or a gambler or a womanizer and all that other crap that I am, you know, or a religious type, tell me about AA. I mean, most people that like AA want you to be there because they are.

Therapist/consultant: Yeah. Well, none of that here. My opinion is that if you don't get involved in a program, and I mean really work the program, you'll be dead in a couple of years at most.

Mr. Thompson: Hmm. Something to consider, I guess. Shit, I got a lot to live for. Well, (sadly) at least I did.

Father Jack: You can get it all back, Gary. Listen to what he's saying.

Therapist/consultant: Maybe. I don't want to promise anything, except to Gary that he might have a better chance if he gets some addictions treatment.

Mr. Thompson finally agreed to go to GA and AA. He maintained sobriety and a gambling free life-style. Eventually, he entered family therapy, although his marriage was not saved. Gerald eventually found a steady job in another state and Lonnie enrolled in college. Mr. Thompson credited the emergency worker's candidness and honesty to saving his life and convincing him that he needed help.

Chapter Eight

Translating Problem Solving into Specific Actions: Empowerment of the Resistant Family

The final phase of the crisis intervention interview is specified by the letter T in our acronym, for the *translation* of the resistant family's experience at problem solving into specific goals. If the therapist/consultant has been fortunate and has done a good job in previous portions of the interview, he or she will find a family system better prepared to move ahead with any solutions that have been generated. However, the family may lack one essential component before it can solve its own problems. It may not know how to apply the generated solutions to its problems in living. Consequently, the family may not believe that any action it implements will effectively solve its problems. Therefore, the family needs to be empowered.

We empower the resistant family by attempting to foster task accomplishment of previously decided upon goals deemed to be helpful for problem solving. In other words, we help the family solve its own problems by showing it how to translate these goals into viable behaviors that impact on the family system's functioning. The principal device that we use for empowerment is the Behavioral Contract, described below. The Behavioral Contract includes *realistic actions the family can perform to decrease the severity of the problems it is experiencing.*

In contrast to earlier phases of the crisis interview, this phase involves almost a complete shift in the role of the therapist toward that of systems consultant. The crisis consultant (formerly the crisis therapist) now attempts to objectively engage the family in a realistic examination of present and future behaviors. The consultant also suggests a number of brief interventions designed to increase the family system's appropriate use of appropriate homeostasis as a crisis buffer. These include the modeling of effective stress coping mechanisms, with special emphasis on increasing the system social support. The goals of these interventions are to augment the present and future ability of the family system to withstand stressors so that it eventually becomes more resilient and less crisis-prone.

The general tone of this portion of the interview is optimistic, yet realistic. The crisis consultant is supportive, hopeful, respectful, and pragmatic. He or she recognizes that the resistant family may not succeed in attempts to solve problems, but nonetheless, must try on their own. Above all, the consultant strives to communicate to the family that they are responsible for their own present and future behavior and that they can succeed if they choose to do so.

Although the consultant is imbuing hope within the family, he or she is also simultaneously sensitizing them to the possibility their immediate actions for solving problems may prove to be frustrating or even futile, at least for the present. The consultant acknowledges the reality of the family's predicament and respectfully empathizes with the severity of suffering it has engendered. He or she realizes that, in spite of the family's efforts, the nature of the problem may be of sufficient severity as to endure for a long period. The consultant tactfully approaches the resistant family regarding this possibility, and reiterates that his/her door is always open if they find it necessary to return and explore other therapeutic options. Options always exist if the family retains hope and begins to develop a sense of self-efficacy regarding potential to change.

THE BEHAVIORAL CONTRACT

The heart of the final portion of the crisis interview, whether it extends over one or many sessions, is the creation of a family Behavioral Contract. Families should always leave the crisis session with mutually negotiated and agreed upon instructions regarding how to manage their present problem. There are several reasons for this. First, most families expect to conclude their session with something tangible, just as anyone who visits a physician usually expects to receive a prescription or other form of treatment. Secondly, families need to feel that they have done something positive and accomplished something tangible as a result of their crisis. Finally, the Behavioral Contract reduces any confusion regarding the family's and consultant's present and future responsibilities.

Based on the family's desired problem-focused solution and the consultant's assessment of the family's needs, the consultant and the family develop specifics of the Behavioral Contract. These include a brief outline of *who* does *what* and *when*. A brief description of how to determine whether the goal or behavior has been accomplished should also be included. Additionally, we believe that the Behavioral Contract should involve at least two components; (a) behavioral monitoring and (b) behavioral initiation. In the Behavioral Contract the family typically agrees to complete a task to accomplish a specific goal. This is the behavioral initiation. However, examination of whether the goal has been reached involves behavioral monitoring. Clearly, the two are highly inter-related. For example, the behavioral injunctive, "Take your son to the emergency room if he gets much worse," implies not only an action, behavioral initiation, but also behavioral monitoring in that the achievement of the goal can be clearly observed. Even the paradoxical intervention, "Don't change anything until we see you on your regular therapy day," involves both initiation and monitoring.

The client family must also be able to monitor which factors in their system remain the same. Behavioral monitoring of this type involves initiating thought and discussion regarding exactly what it is that is not being changed. A similar paradox involves the injunction, "Don't do anything, but monitor the situation closely." The more closely family members monitor the situation, the more they can intervene in their own system.

Although not always possible to obtain, a formal, written Behavioral Contract is preferred over a verbal agreement, especially with resistant families. Agreements in writing are more inviolate and less apt to cause later disagreement on what family members really meant or stated. Our goal, for both therapeutic and legal reasons, is to obtain everything in writing and include it as part of the treatment record. Optimally, each family member's role in crisis management should be articulated in detail. Contingency procedures should be included in case the family or any member does not abide by the contract. An emergency number should be provided for additional intervention if necessary. Ideally, each family member should also receive and sign a copy of the Behavioral Contract.

Table 8.1 is a copy of a Behavioral Contract signed by a resistant family. The family involved has a history of being both treatment resistant and crisis-prone. Note the details that are provided, most of which will be discussed below. It is often best to use a personal computer and generate a number of narrative shells (or models) specific to a variety of common crises. For example, we are aware of one crisis center that has constructed a series of macros for a popular word processing program. Using the shell as a guideline, the therapist and the family conjointly and quickly construct a Behavioral Contract. A copy of the contract should also be made available at all times to other therapists in the facility who may encounter the family during an emergency.

TABLE 8.1. Behavioral Contract

Family Contract between the family and Dr. Johnson.

1. John has agreed to take his medications in front of Lisa in the morning and in the evening, for the next month. Lisa agrees to get the prescription refilled.
2. Because John and Mom are fighting too often, Mom agrees to meet with John on Tuesday and Thursday for one hour for "nonfighting" time. During this time no one will raise voices or say anything negative about the other. They are free to talk about anything else. Both John and Mom must be straight during this time.
3. Because family communications are poor, Cyndi agrees to chair a family communications meeting, once a week on Wednesday nights. The family will talk about common problems they are having and things they are feeling. During this meeting, the same rules that apply in Dr. Johnson's office will apply. This means no swearing and no interrupting of someone else. No one may drink during this session.
4. John has agreed to call the mental health center today to discuss resuming treatment. Lisa will help John do this. John will also tell them that he has stopped his medication on his own and is just restarting today.

5. Mom agrees to have Natasha write down the number of drinks Mom drinks and cigarettes she smokes each week. Natasha will get this information on a daily basis and will post it on the refrigerator for the family to see.
6. John will call Dr. Johnson once a week, on Wednesday morning, until he can get a regular appointment at the mental health center.
7. Dr. Johnson will call the family at least once a week to see how they are doing. The family agrees to come in again if Dr. Johnson believes they should.
8. Natasha, Cyndi, Lisa, and John all agree to go to Al Anon at least once a week for the next month. John will call and find out where meetings are held.
9. Mom agrees that if she does continue drinking she will not raiser her voice at anyone in the house after she has had a drink. Nor will she try to correct or discipline any of the children after she has been drinking.
10. If at any time Mom decides she wants to quit drinking, she will call Dr. Johnson who will discuss the options with her. She also agrees to try AA again. Cyndi will call the AA and get transportation.
11. John agrees to stay out of Cyndi's room and also to use headphones when listening to music at all times. Natasha agrees to monitor this for the two. If he can do this for one month, Mom agrees to let John buy the CD player he has been saving for.

By signing below, you indicate that you agree to these terms.

INTEGRATING FAMILY ASSESSMENT INTO THE BEHAVIORAL CONTRACT

In Chapter Six we stated that it is critical to evaluate the family according to both their crisis-proneness and treatment resistance. We now wish to use this information to help families "operationalize" their goals. It is countertherapeutic to prescribe goals that a family realistically cannot or will not perform. Such an action only serves to demoralize families and convince them that their stresses are uncontrollable. Consequently, any interventions with the family are tempered by the reality of the family's present problems and past history.

Table 8.2 illustrates the possible combinations of crisis-proneness and treatment resistance, and summarizes our recommenda-

TABLE 8.2. Crisis-Proneness, Treatment Resistance, and Treatment Recommendations

DEGREE OF FAMILY CRISIS-PRONESS (Number of Crises per Year)	DEGREE OF FAMILY TREATMENT RESISTANCE	CRISIS MANAGEMENT RECOMMENDATIONS
Mild (1-4)	*Mild* (1-2)	Family usually needs minimal intervention.
Mild-Moderate (5-8)	*Moderate* (3-4)	Family can usually handle most crises with minimal post session therapist intervention. Usually can meet goals of Behavioral Contract.
Mild-Moderate (9-14)	*Moderate-Severe* (5-7)	Family likely to terminate once crisis is over. Family will need additional supervision and monitoring contact to keep it motivated and to ensure that it follows up on treatment recommendations. Consider use of link therapist and outside social or family resourses.
Moderate-Severe (14-20)	*Mild-Moderate* (5-7)	Family likely to return in crisis. Will need frequent contact to reassure it that it can succeed. Usually will meet terms of Behavioral Contract if consultant is encouraging and optimistic.
Moderate-Severe (> 20)	*Moderate-Severe* (5-7)	Classic high risk family. Will need frequent monitoring *and* reassurance.

tions regarding behavioral tasks associated with these groups. Notice that as crisis-proneness and treatment resistance increase, the type of recommendations for the family change. In general, treatment resistant families require an increase in *monitoring* interventions by the consultant to ascertain whether they are performing the appropriate problem-solving tasks. Such interventions are designed to increase the family's motivation to continue the desired behaviors. On the other hand, crisis-prone families need *more frequent feedback* regarding the efficacy of their interventions, since they are more likely to be overcome by stressors and easily discouraged when change is slow.

When families present with a moderate degree of crisis-proneness (three to four on our scale) and treatment resistance they can usually be entrusted to carry out any behavioral tasks agreed upon with the consultant. The Behavioral Contract can make use of the fact that such families are often excellent managers of their own symptoms. As long as these families are sufficiently empowered to solve their problems they can usually do so, although they may lack appropriate skills.

However, as a family's crisis-prone score increases, so does the likelihood that the family will return with a future–and unrelated– problem. When families are crisis-prone (five to seven on our scale) but not treatment resistant, they usually can carry out mutually agreed upon problem-focused objectives, but only with support and reassurance from the therapist. The Behavioral Contract should include provisions for the fact the consultant may have to make numerous contacts with the client family to ensure compliance with recommendations. These families typically possess little sense of control over their situation and may require more frequent contact than the therapist wishes. Nevertheless, their prognosis is good. If handled correctly, the crisis will be a genuine growth experience, as the family learns it can manage the extreme stress and still survive.

The degree of past treatment compliance ascertained during the evaluation portion of the crisis session can be taken as a rough estimate of the likelihood the family will follow through with stated goals. Therefore, we have found it crucial to assume that families with a history of not being treatment compliant (five, six, or seven on our scale) *cannot* be consistently entrusted to complete the tasks agreed upon during the crisis session. Therefore, the Behavioral

Contract for these families should not rely exclusively upon familial monitoring of behavior or any other possible actions in which the family might be noncompliant. This includes the monitoring of the mental status of family members.

Furthermore, it is not uncommon for these families to drop out of treatment, even when a family member is psychotic or suicidal. The major technique useful for keeping treatment resistant families involved during a crisis is frequent contact. It may be necessary for the consultant to incorporate daily calls to such families into the Behavioral Contract. Other extended family or community resources can be employed in the contract to "check in" with these families during crisis periods. Unfortunately, frequent contact has less effect in convincing such systems of the need to consider longer-term therapy beyond the crisis session.

When families score a six or, especially, a seven on our scale of treatment compliance, it is often helpful to temporarily abandon attempts to foster family behavior and instead encourage responsible individuals within the family system to engage in needed action. For example, if the family's goal is to monitor a schizophrenic adolescent, the therapist/consultant might wish to assign this task to one particular family member with demonstrated potential for responsibility. We do not wish to do this for very long. Otherwise, families will absorb the message that their collective behavior can be redeemed by one or more responsible family members. Such families will also rather quickly sabotage efforts of the most functional member. However, in serious crisis situations, the treatment resistant family is often more likely to carry out its required tasks when they are assigned to individual members. This will be addressed later, below, in our discussion regarding link therapists.

Obviously, the most difficult families in crisis are true resistant systems: those that score five or more on each of our two scales. Such families generally have to be *seen* at frequent intervals during the crisis to first ensure they possess the necessary self-efficacy to complete agreed upon tasks. Secondly, frequent contacts ensure they do not lose interest in solving their problems. Potential need for frequent contact should be specified in the Behavioral Contract. Telephone management of such families may also be insufficient and the consultant should allot sufficient time for face-to-face interaction, if necessary. Often, several revisions of the Behavioral Contract will need to be negotiated for these types of families, depending upon the ongoing behaviors of various members.

SPECIFICS OF THE BEHAVIORAL CONTRACT: INTERVENTIONS TO CHANGE DYSFUNCTIONAL COPING

Earlier we highlighted the fact that resistant families display a significant amount of dysfunctional coping, perhaps because such coping typically serves to return the family system to homeostasis, at least temporarily. However, over longer periods, dysfunctional coping styles tend to perpetuate family dysfunction. To the family, poor coping strategies fulfill an important need of providing systemic stabilization during crises. Unfortunately, resolution of the crisis does not improve effectiveness of dysfunctional coping mechanisms, and the family is prone to repeated crises at a later date.

Clinical experience has suggested that rapid and permanent changes in family coping are often possible for the resistant family *if these changes are adopted during crisis situations*. Clinicians who have followed the "roller coaster model" of family stress have long known this. Chaos theory now provides a clearer model of how permanent changes can follow stress. The response to crises often involves a willingness to try new behaviors. Behavioral changes instituted in response to life crises are more likely to be maintained, simply because they are so rewarding. Hence, the family crisis is an excellent window of opportunity to help the family learn more effective coping strategies.

Consequently, we incorporate our previous assessment of the family's coping weaknesses and strengths into the Behavioral Contract. We then suggest *alternate coping skills* that can be more helpful than the family's present coping methods, giving the family specific examples. Many of these alternatives are based upon the popular use of extra-session family meetings designed to increase both functional coping and family interaction.

Identification of the Stressor

Families that cannot identify problems are not as troubled by them initially as families acutely aware of their problems. However, this lack of awareness is only temporary, since unidentifiable problems eventually produce more uncontrollable life situations. Unfortunately, denial of family stressors is often a problem best undertaken in long-term therapy, rather than in brief crisis intervention.

One useful method for increasing realization of current stressors involves ongoing family sessions designed to help each of the family members identify "What's bothering our family?" While this may be moderately effective within the office, it is often most effective when conducted at home. As a "homework" assignment, families can be instructed to hold meetings once or twice a week to identify all of their present stressors. Each family member can be encouraged to separately write down their thoughts and feelings regarding family difficulties. Then, either with the consultant or at home, the family should compare and discuss these sentiments.

This often results in a greater awareness of stressors that are present in the system. It is important the consultant consistently emphasize the seriousness of this meeting, as some families are apt to take such a novel request somewhat flippantly. Formal notes of this meeting can be taken by a family "secretary"; preferably, an adolescent who otherwise might not feel as involved. Minutes from the family meeting should be reported to the consultant, if the family is continuing in treatment, and be made part of the treatment records. When combined with the following two considerations below, family sessions are especially effective in getting families in crisis to recognize they have significant *family* stressors.

Locus of the Problem

This area of dysfunctional coping assessment concerns the answer to the following question: When a problem exists at home, is it considered a family or an individual problem? When families have difficulty accepting a family-oriented locus of problem behaviors, they are much less likely to be treatment compliant. In these cases family members are encouraged in their Behavioral Contract to discuss the *causes* of problems together at a family meeting, with all members present. This fosters shifting the locus of the problem from the individual to the family. Usually, the family is able to recognize the family locus of the problem much more quickly than it is able to recognize its many stressors. Typically, only one family meeting will be required for this topic, whereas several ongoing meetings may be necessary to enable families to understand the stresses in their lives.

Approach to the Problem

As stated in Chapter Five, dysfunctional coping in this area involves the family's general orientation to solving problems. If the consultant has determined that families have coping deficits in this area, the Behavioral Contract can include provisions to foster family problem solving. For example, after identifying difficulties, family members can be encouraged to mutually discuss solutions to future problems in a forum that involves and includes the entire family. Usually, the family meeting is the best vehicle for this, but a session with a consultant may also be appropriate.

The family's previous experience with the therapist/consultant can serve as a model for the fact that they can indeed work together to generate solutions. Families are empowered when the therapist gently reiterates to them that any successes accomplished in the therapist's office can be duplicated at home.

Families with severe deficits in problem solving may need additional and specific training in this area that is more in the domain of therapy than consultation or crisis intervention. We recommend the methods of Shure and her associates, (e.g., Shure, 1992a; 1992b; 1992c), who have provided detailed scripts for teaching problem-solving skills to young people, parents, and families.[1] For example, some severely impaired families can also benefit from working together to solve games or T.V. quiz shows. This type of homework assignment can usually be incorporated into a Behavioral Contract. The family's success in this prescribed nightly behavior can often be generalized to other and more important situations.

Tolerance of Others

Paranoid, hostile families are invariably treatment resistant. Perhaps this is because they often isolate themselves from others outside of the family who could provide corrective feedback regarding their behavior and attitudes. Unfortunately, tolerance of others out-side of the family is one of the most difficult stress coping skills to foster during a crisis situation. The Adlerian solution of encourag-ing intolerant people to volunteer to help those less fortunate may be effective in some situations and can be incorporated into a Be-havioral Contract. Behavioral solutions which discourage negative verbalization regarding others can also be helpful, but often are sabotaged outside of the consultant's office.

Family Affection

Families lacking in affection do not interact well, and hence do not share their troubles. As a result, while specific individuals may be clearly pathological, the family system as an entity appears more stable than it actually is. To break this cycle we wish to increase family displays of affection, especially during periods of crisis.

The incorporation of ongoing family meetings into the Behavior-al Contract may automatically engender an increase in family affec-tion. Also, temporary increases in family displays of affection may be gained by mere suggestion. However, once increased rates of affection are encountered, families are likely to generate hostility when those rates return to baseline. This seems especially true regarding resistant couples with histories of infidelity or abuse. Hence, care must be taken with this method.

Asking family members to reward each other on a more frequent basis–either with words or specific behaviors–is often extraordi-narily helpful for increasing family trust and mutual affection. For example, Stuart (1980) advocates the technique of "caring days" to boost commitment to a troubled marriage. Similar techniques have been successfully incorporated into Behavioral Contracts of resis-tant families with a consequent increase in family affection. Sur-prisingly, the technique seems to work as well for "neutral" family members as it does for those with constant conflict. When con-flictual parties in a family system can agree to reinforce each other on a daily basis, the conflict is often contained and genuine displays of spontaneous affection may increase. These positive displays often generalize and are maintained long past the expiration of the Behavioral Contract.

Communication Utilization

The lack of family communication exacerbates almost any crisis. Families instinctively know this, but often lack the practice and skills for effective communication. Weekly "communications sessions"–a variety of the family meeting advocated above–that include all family members are effective in increasing communications and can be easily prescribed in the Behavioral Contract. During these sessions families should be instructed to talk about everything, not just their problems. Resistant families can usually employ such sessions for up to three or four weeks at a time before they lose interest.

Many writers of various family therapy orientations (e.g., Haley, 1976, 1980; Stuart, 1980) indicate that dysfunctional couples or families lack fundamental and basic communications skills. Communications problems are common in well over three-quarters of resistant families and do *not* typically resolve spontaneously. However, they may, in some cases, ameliorate themselves when other systemic factors improve. Despite this, chronically poor communications skills may remain one of the many factors that perpetuates poor family system functioning and crisis-proneness. Communications skills can be successfully taught, using any number of strategies available in the literature. In our experience, resistant families that eschew therapy may be quite agreeable to receiving conjoint or group "communications training" and often show substantial benefits from this type of intervention.

Family Cohesion

Family cohesion is assessed, in part, by asking "When something bad happens at home does your family stick together?" Family cohesion is one of the most difficult coping variables to directly alter, especially over the short term. Regardless, attempts are common in structural/strategic therapies (e.g., Haley, 1980), and often succeed. On the other hand, when applied to families that are likely to drop out of treatment, such interventions may make the family worse, with no chance for the therapist to correct this damage later. Specifically, behavioral interventions designed to increase family cohesion often creates extra tension in the home. This, in turn, can cause deterioration in other aspects of the system's functioning. Unless a therapist is able to intervene over a longer period to correct these potential deteriorations, the resistant family can get worse from attempts to increase family cohesion. Consequently, we generally prefer to indirectly increase family cohesion through the use of family meetings, increased social supports, and resource utilization, discussed at length below.

Family Roles

As structural therapists have long known, family roles can be changed through family therapy. And, as strategic therapists have known, this can be done relatively quickly. Unfortunately, resistant families often display a tendency to revert to former dysfunctional roles with the passage of time and cessation of the family crisis. The systemic pressures the resistant family exerts are likely to cause a "spontaneous recovery" of former behaviors. Thus, although the consultant may suggest changes in family roles during crises, it is unlikely the high risk family will maintain these changes for very long. However, it may be worth a try.

Paradoxical interventions to change family roles may be more effective for resistant families. For example, in a family where the father classically undermines the mother's authority, the therapist can state the following: "Well, I think your family would have less problems if Dad and Mom were more consistent with the children. But this is much too difficult of a change for your family to make and may take many years to complete." Sometimes interventions such as these will cause the family to move in the desired direction, just to prove the therapist wrong. Paradoxical interventions are also useful, inasmuch as lack of success will not further demoralize the family and contribute to its sense of hopelessness.

Resource Utilization

Improvement in resource utilization is the most effective change the consultant can suggest for the resistant family. The most common method for increasing resource utilization is to encourage increased interaction with other, *non-nuclear*, family members. Behavioral Contracts often involve provisions for increased contact with other family members. We are not completely optimistic about this method inasmuch as high risk families often have family of origin systems that may be equally dysfunctional. For example, Johnson (1989) found that spouse abusers have adequate social networks, as judged by their sizes. Unfortunately, these networks are predominantly composed of other family members, many of whom may hold the same dysfunctional values as the abusers and may tolerate and even encourage ongoing abuse.

A second method of enhancing social support with resistant families is to encourage participation in religious or community groups. Religious institutions are sometimes deliberately avoided by family therapists who believe families will simply substitute one treatment provider for another. In general, we disagree with this negative assessment. Religious beliefs can increase a family's perceived ability to control a situation, thereby decreasing crisis-proneness. This is especially useful for high risk families. However, religion is usually not the panacea that some clients believe it to be and under certain circumstances can decrease a family's desire to make healthy changes. Therapists who confront these problems with client families can pursue a number of options. Perhaps the best is to seek consultation with colleagues whose religious background is similar to that of the clients being treated. Often, it is helpful to contact a sympathetic member of the clergy and seek advice. Counselors affiliated with seminaries or other religious institutions similar to the client family's can also be extremely helpful.

Similar to religious groups in their capacity to enhance social support are the numerous self-help modalities that are popular across the world. Self-help treatment remains the first line of defense for a variety of addiction disorders (McCown & Johnson, 1992b). Self-help groups, especially Twelve-Step-oriented groups, are perceived to be highly successful in the treatment of substance abuse. Treatment typically consists of a systematic and relatively unvaried progression through a program designed to rehabilitate the substance abuser, prescribing a common approach to recovery and emphasizing commonalities of substance abuse.

Twelve-Step groups, and to a lesser extent other self-help groups, offer the individual immediate and 24-hour access to social support. Appropriate feedback potentially lacking in the individual's family or network is replaced by a worldwide community of supportive peer counselors. From our perspective, Twelve-Step groups are even more useful inasmuch as they accept failure of members in a relatively nonjudgmental fashion and ultimately empower the individual.

Until recently, many family therapists were typically reluctant to recommend self-help to families. One reason for this reluctance centered upon concern regarding symptom substitution–substituting one sick system for another. Along with this, they worried–often correctly–that self-help groups did not adequately address underlying problems in family pathology. Many therapists can provide a plethora of examples regarding family systems that remain pathological despite involvement in AA, Al Anon, or other organizations. Although self-help group members have long implicated family dynamics as an integral part of the recovery process, many have also been suspicious of family therapists. However, during the past ten years this has changed rather dramatically and it is now common for individuals to be involved in both types of treatment.

Self-help, like religion, is not a panacea for the resistant family. Self-help is a serious approach for any disorder characterized by crisis-proneness and difficulty in engaging in treatment. Recommendation and referral is not to be made lightly, since it involves many life-style changes. Self-help works brilliantly well for some families, less well with others, and fails for an undetermined number of systems. Our research group has sought to establish optimal circumstances facilitating self-help group efficacy. For example, impulsive people often experience difficulty in Twelve-Step groups, probably because they do not attend regularly (McCown, 1990). The best–and perhaps the only–predictor of how effective self-help is perceived to be lies in the opinion of the family that tries it. Of course, individual family members often have different reactions. For example, one member may find self-help approaches to be particularly useful, while others find them to be a waste of time.

Unpublished data we have collected regarding resistant families suggests that for approximately 15 percent of such families self-help causes dramatic and positive results *regardless of the problem for which it was prescribed*. Another 10 percent of families make moderate or intermittent use of self-help. An undetermined percentage of families initially reject self-help intervention, yet turn to it when therapy is terminated. About 5 percent of families made sporadic or periodic use of self-help as a form of crisis intervention. Clearly, any treatment helpful to at least a third of resistant families is worth pursuing and should be considered as an option to be incorporated into the Behavioral Contract.

Violence

As long as violence is a transitory and crisis-limited phenomena, our clinical impression is that it *can often* be interrupted in the resistant family. The spouse or lover with a rare or intermittent history of violence is less likely to repeat, except under conditions of extreme stress including the stress of substance use. When families with mild histories of violence quit hitting, they usually start talking. A "no violence" provision in the Behavioral Contract can often stop such violence with ensuing positive impact on the family system.

However, the longer violence has been used as a coping mechanism, the less likely brief interventions will be effective. Perhaps more importantly, the more routine the violence has become, the more likely it is to be intractable. Family members seem to become simultaneously "addicted" to its occurrence and immune to its deviance. Furthermore, the cessation of violence may often result in a decrease in family functioning in other domains. In general, chronic domestic violence is an exceedingly serious problem that rarely responds to brief interventions. The problem is even more difficult to treat in families that are treatment resistant.

When violence involves consenting adults, our position is that the involved parties should make the decision regarding its tolerance. If people involved in a battering relationship pursue and continue this behavior, it is ultimately their own responsibility and choice. This position is certainly controversial, but we believe it reflects clinical reality. To reiterate a central theme of this book, clients cannot be saved from themselves against their wills. They can, however, be empowered to make informed decisions. If these clients choose to end or modify battering relationships, they should be offered every option available, including shelter, individual and group counseling, and family treatment. If key family members are not interested in treatment, aggressive empowerment of family members willing to change should proceed through appropriate referral to agencies or therapists experienced in treating violent systems.

On the other hand, violence and sexual abuse toward those incapable of responsible behaviors or choices must be stopped immediately. Such behavior is never appropriate. The therapist must make this clear from the onset and communicate this directly to the family. The Behavioral Contract should also specify this. Furthermore, the consultant should provide clear consequences to continued violence in the Behavioral Contract.

Nonprescription Drugs and Alcohol

As Steinglass' (1977) research has shown, alcohol consumption, despite its latent dysfunctionality, often serves an important family function. Attempts to abruptly stop resistant family members from drinking, especially without additional community supports or ongoing therapy, are rarely effective. Sometimes such attempts pose even greater difficulty inasmuch as the family system often experiences immediate deterioration following such a dramatic change. For example, an anxious, poorly skilled mother might stop drinking, and yet begin to verbally abuse her children. When therapy is ongoing, behavioral changes such as these can be monitored. But when the family is unlikely to return for additional treatment, abrupt and unsupervised cessation of substance use can portend danger to other system members.

However, since excessive drug and alcohol abuse yields such negative consequences, the family should be always be confronted when excessive use is suspected. Since substance abuse is frequently a product of dysfunctional attempts to cope with stress, consultants should not hesitate to assess for and suggest substance abuse as one of the family's problems. Appropriate referral for treatment, both professional and self-help, should be politely but firmly made in these circumstances, even to the most resistant family.

Alcohol and drug usage are chronic problems. Abrupt cessation of this coping mechanism may increase family crisis-proneness (Kaufman, 1985). Often, addictions professionals overlook this and believe that brief interventions can ameliorate these problems. Consequently, they tend to "come down hard" in a confrontational manner on any family member who abuses drugs or alcohol, despite the family dynamics involved. Although these techniques may prove effective for individuals or in cases where the IP presents with a substance abuse problem, they do not necessarily work well when substances are used as a coping mechanism. Nor are they particularly helpful for treatment resistant systems.

One technique that is often effective lies in suggesting that the substance abusing family attempt to refrain from substance use and to report back to the consultant if they cannot. When the family returns to this dysfunctional method of coping–which they almost always do–the need for more extensive therapy and/or self-help involvement becomes more evident and can then be highlighted. In this manner blame can be avoided and the family can begin to take responsibility for its own substance usage. Eventually, resistance can be weakened sufficiently and real change becomes possible.

IDENTIFICATION OF POTENTIAL COMPLIANCE PROBLEMS

Prior to finalizing a Behavioral Contract, the consultant should help the resistant family identify and overcome difficulties that might interfere with their problem-solving goals. The first barrier the family typically encounters is a lack of necessary skills to implement their solution to a problem. For example, a family may decide the optimal way to manage an adolescent daughter's rebelliousness lies in appropriate limit setting. This may be something they have relatively little experience in implementing. One helpful strategy used to demonstrate and impart such skills involves the use of role play.

During the 1970s and early 1980s role playing was a common therapeutic adjunct, credited with a variety of therapeutic benefits and practical advantages. However, the use of role playing has declined in popularity recently, perhaps because some practitioners consider it "artificial," or too time consuming. Nevertheless, role playing remains a good method of helping families cope with stressors likely to be encountered outside of the therapeutic office or emergency room. Family Study 8.1, below, illustrates how role playing can be effective with resistant families.

Family Study 8.1. The Smiths

  Lisa and John Smith, 47 and 44, were unable to set limits on their adolescent daughter Leslie, 15. The adolescent was allowed to determine her own hours and responsibilities within the family, and was frequently in trouble with the police or school officials. This would prompt a family crisis. The family would terminate therapy after a few sessions, convinced the problem was solved. Invariably, the cycle would repeat.

  Upon interviewing the parents, the therapist realized that neither Mr. or Mrs. Smith could consistently tell their daughter "No." The daughter would usually succeed in haranguing them until she got her way. The therapist suspected that this might be due to the parents' longstanding needs to be loved, based upon their own families of origin. The system was faced with the immediate need to set limits on Leslie, a need that could not wait for the effects of longer-term therapy.

  The therapist decided to spend half of the family's crisis session role playing with the mother and father on effective limit-setting with their daughter. The therapist questioned and cajoled the family for over an hour, attempting to teach them to be comfortable with providing discipline. Although the family felt extremely uncomfortable with this intervention, they generally cooperated through practicing the appropriate techniques. They incorporated limit setting into a Behavioral Contract and were able to employ this skill successfully with their daughter the next time she tested the family limits.

We have also found it helpful to encourage the family to role play outside of the crisis evaluation setting, especially in their own home. Along these lines, a useful component of the Behavioral

Contract involves time outside of sessions designated for role playing, usually on a daily basis. Some resistant families will terminate this practice abruptly, but usually not before they have sufficiently mastered the necessary skills.

A second method of fostering task accomplishment involves the role of the consultant as an executive organizer for the client family. Inasmuch as the resistant family is often stymied by simple obstacles, the consultant needs to evaluate their potential plan of action and question the family on various options to pursue if certain predictable roadblocks emerge. The consultant can then use his or her experience, judgment, and ability to help the family predict such impediments and plan viable ways to maneuver around them. Often, we refer to this technique as "Mine Clearing" and it is illustrated in Family Study 8.2 below, a lengthy account of a crisis intervention session involving a violent racist.

Family Study 8.2. Mr. Boudreaux

Mr. Boudreaux, age 22, was a rural Louisiana man of Cajun descent. He approached the local mental health center because of fears that he would physically harm his estranged wife, Tammy, 20. Tammy had recently left "Mr. B.," as his friends call him, for a flamboyant older man from their tiny Louisiana town. This man was known by the moniker of "Kingfish," after the famed former Governor Huey Long. Mr. B. was livid and stated that he wanted to kill Kingfish. The situation was exacerbated by the fact that Kingfish was African-American in origin, and Mr. B. was intolerant of interracial relationships.

An evaluation determined that Mr. B. was probably not an immediate risk to anyone as long as he remained sober. However, once he started drinking he would likely become violent. Recently, he had threatened Kingfish three times, each of which occurred when they were both drunk. Unfortunately for all involved, drinking was an integral part of the subculture to which Mr. B. belonged. In this small town it was inevitable that Kingfish and Mr. B. would run across each other, and do so while they were both inebriated.

The crisis therapist, now acting in a consultational role, was appropriately concerned. Racial tensions were running high in the small town. Furthermore, the client had a history of violence and possessed several guns. Apart from some equally racist friends and a dysfunctional family, he had few social supports.

Initially the consultant suggested a trial of disulfiram, so that any episodes of drinking would lead to physical discomfort. Mr. B. rejected this idea and stated instead that he would confine himself to taverns in the portion of town where he would not likely encounter Kingfish "or any other nigger." The consultant then suggested they try some anticipation of potential problems.

Consultant: So what will you do if you do run into him?

Mr. B.: I won't. I won't run into him. I told you, I don't go to nigger bars.

Consultant: Okay. So you don't. But what will happen if you do?

Mr. B.: I won't. I swear. Ain't no nigger that's worth me going to jail for. And the way the judges are around here, you kill a nigger, and you're in jail for life. Fuck that! Pardon my French.

Consultant: I believe you. You've been very honest with me. But what if you get drunk and start looking for trouble?

Mr. B.: I won't go after him.

Consultant: Wait a minute. Now you told me already that three times this month you got drunk and threatened Kingfish. Right?

Mr. B.: Yup.

Consultant: Now what will happen if you get drunk again?

Mr. B.: Hmmm. I didn't think of that. Holy shit! Once I get fired up, no telling what I might do.

Consultant: So maybe you shouldn't drink at all for a while, at least until this blows over. Until you feel more in control . . . Let's get some of this down on paper, so that we all agree.

Mr. B.: No . . . . Well, I don't know. (long pause) You might be right. Maybe I could take the drinking pill (disulfiram) and tell them that my doctor told me not to drink. I could live with that. Give my liver a rest.

Later in the session, Mr. B. states that some of his friends have been encouraging him to "cut up some niggers." The therapist explores this with the client and attempts to help the client plan accordingly.

Consultant: So what will happen if you run across Oscar or Lafitte or any of those guys? You know, and they start talking to you about going out and creating some trouble with some blacks? Got any ideas what to do then?

Mr. B.: I ain't got anything against any nigger but Kingfish. I'll tell them that. To me, I don't care what color you are as long as you don't fuck with me. That's what my mama taught me.

Consultant: What if your friends give you a load of shit? You know, tell you that you're chicken? Can you hear that? "Mr. B's a chicken!"

Mr. B.: If anyone tells Mr. B. he's chicken, they know they have a fight on their hands. No one fucks with Mr. B. I'll show them who's chickshit! I bust 'em up on the head! Pop! Pow!

Consultant: So you fight your friends instead of Kingfish. Hmmm. I am a bit confused. Won't that land you in Angola (the state jail)? I thought that was one of your goals—to avoid any more problems with the law.

Mr. B.: Not if I don't cut 'em up bad! (laughs). No, I see. I should be prepared for some shit. I can take it. I'm a strong man.

Consultant: I don't doubt that. But I'm a little worried. What if you run across Kingfish somewhere? You know, like on the bayou fishing? You told me that when you aren't ready for things, sometimes you overreact, remember?

Mr. B.: Yeah . . . You know, I could see my guys setting me up on a little fishing trip, just to watch the fireworks. I'd land in Angola for sure. Man, I would sure miss fishing in prison (laughing). I might have my gun with me and bam! One dead nigger.

Consultant: So maybe you need to turn your guns over to someone? For a while, at least. Would you agree to put that in a contract with me?

Mr. B.: Alright. I won't go to Bayou _____. That's by his sister's. There's a good chance I would run into him, 'cause he likes to crab and they're running good now. Running the best they run in a couple years. Your husband like to crab? I could show him some fine spots. I got my traps up from here to Thibodeaux.

Consultant: (ignoring the diversion). And your guns? The handguns, anyhow. I want you to sign our contract saying you'll put them where you can't get them.

Mr. B.: I'll give 'em to my daddy. At least until I feel less angry. Maybe for a few days.

Consultant: Okay, why don't you call your dad and make arrangements? Then we can put some of this in our contract, so it's clear to everyone.

Mr. B.: Okay. He's got to pick me up anyhow.

The above transcript also illustrates the necessity of the systems therapist to rise above his or her values and communicate effectively within the client system. In this case the therapist had an appropriate revulsion regarding the client's racial values and intolerance. However, she did not try to foster a more liberal worldview on the client or his system, but instead worked with him to solve the problem at hand.

During behavioral rehearsals, such as the one above, it is also helpful to give families in crisis some alternative strategies to try in case their primary means of coping fails. Usually phrases such as "You might also try . . ." or "You might even consider . . ." are both innocuous and effective. Alternative strategies should be presented within the context of the client system's previously generated solutions. For example, if a client family has stated that they intend to solve their financial problems primarily by borrowing from relatives, the consultant could also suggest that they seek state assistance or general relief. If time permits, role playing should include alternative strategies. If not, the crisis consultant should make it clear who can assist the family in pursuing alternative courses should they be deemed appropriate. Family Study 8.3 exhibits the importance of therapeutic assistance in generation of options and alternative plans of action.

Family Study 8.3. The Washingtons

John and Wanda Washington were a resistant family with a son who was a crack cocaine abuser. With the help of an emergency therapist, the couple was able to generate a potential plan of action for treatment of their son. This involved seeking inpatient treatment for their son the next time he returned home.

Although the family was convinced that their resolute decision would solve the problem, the therapist insisted that they generate at least three other courses of action in case hospitalization proved an unviable solution. The family reluctantly agreed and incorporated these options into their Behavioral Contract. This came in use, however, when they found that their insurance would not cover their son.

SUBSYSTEMS THERAPY: LINK THERAPISTS AND THE BEHAVIORAL CONTRACT

When it is not possible to engage the entire family system successfully, or to have them implement potential terms of the Behavioral Contract, it is often advantageous to target a specific person within the family to facilitate change. Landau-Stanton and her associates (Landau-Stanton, Griffiths, & Mason, 1982; Landau-Stanton, 1990) discuss family systems undergoing cultural transition and advocate the use of "Link Therapists." A Link Therapist is a member of the family possessing sufficient ego strength to support the family, and simultaneously serve as a quasi-family therapist for the rest of the system. Landau-Stanton (1990) highlights the major requirements for a link, or as we sometimes also call them, liaison therapist. He or she should be a person in the system who has access to all of the subsystems. He or she should also be cooperative with treatment, perhaps one of the more cooperative members of the system. A more in-depth and extensive discussion of the use of link therapists, particularly regarding families in cultural transition, is provided in Landau-Stanton (1990).

In successful link therapy a specific family member can serve as cotherapist and attempt to work directly with other family members within the session and at home. Link therapists may be essential for carrying out specific critical interventions when other family members are less trustworthy. For example, the link therapist can be placed in charge of monitoring a schizophrenic's medication compliance and maintaining an adequate supply of needed psychotropics in the household. We have found that link therapists are also effective if instructed in teaching various cognitive behavioral and behavioral techniques to other family members. Such techniques include cognitive problem solving, behavioral stress reduction, application of contingencies of reinforcement, and monitoring of negative cognitions of various family members. (Therapists without exposure to these areas may wish to request the assistance of more behavioral colleagues). Table 8.2 below summarizes some of the areas we have found link therapists beneficial in working with the resistant family.

TABLE 8.2. Some Uses of Link Therapies with Resistant Families

- Challenging family's negative or hopeless cognitions or verbalizations.
- Coordinating communication with consultant regarding family status.
- Coordinating family meetings or other family sessions.
- Defusing crises in the home.
- Empowering family members with least power in system.
- Exposing family members to stressful topics to reduce family avoidance or to extinguish fear response.
- Implementing "Time Out" to family members under influence of drugs or alcohol.
- Implementing "Time Out" when family members are inappropriate to each other.
- Making and being in charge of keeping therapy appointments.

- Modeling use of outside resources, such as Al Anon or church attendance.
- Monitoring of family members' symptoms, including depression, substance use, and thought disorders.
- Monitoring levels of family stress.
- Organizing leisure activities for family.
- Problem solving with the family.
- Rewarding agreed upon behavior in other family members.
- Teaching relaxation skills to family members.
- Teaching communications skills to family members.
- Teaching assertiveness to family members.
- Teaching problem solving to family members.

The disadvantages of link therapy are that if done poorly, it becomes only an exercise in providing individual therapy and ignores the needs of the rest of the family. Another problem with link therapy is that it may encourage "splitting" and send the resistant family the message that only one member needs to be responsible for family functioning. Family members may also resent that a specific person in the system gets entrusted with major responsibilities. The solution for some of these problems–borrowed from our strategic family therapy colleagues–is to assign a variety of tasks to diverse family members, with the key ones assigned to individuals in the family system who are most likely to complete them.

An example of use of a link therapist for a severely impaired system is presented below. The Kirkpatrick family is a typical example of a chronically crisis-prone and treatment resistant family. In a recent three-month period, members of the Kirkpatrick family made twelve crisis-oriented calls to the police, a private therapist, and a community mental health center.

Family Study 8.4. The Kirkpatricks

Edwin and Molly Kirkpatrick, both 46 years old, are parents from a retired military family. While on active duty in Asia as a helicopter repairman, Sergeant Kirkpatrick was absent from the family for several years. Upon retirement from the service, he was able to obtain a lucrative job repairing helicopters for an oil company. The family then moved from their small mobile home in the North to a comfortable suburb in a Gulf coast city.

Molly Kirkpatrick is a homemaker who has only recently taken a full-time job outside of the house. Presently, she is working as a secretary. She has had two job changes in the past few months. For years, Edwin refused to allow Molly to work "outside," telling her it was "undignified" for a woman to be employed as anything but a "genuine American housewife." After years of complaining that she was "bored silly," Molly finally convinced her husband to allow her to take a paying job.

Edwin and Molly have four children: Edwin, Jr., 24, Donna, 22, Sarah, 19, and Ryan, 13. Upon purchasing the family's new home, both parents encouraged the first three children–who had previously left their parents' residence–to come South and live in the new house. According to Molly, this was because "we have so much room we don't know what to do with it." Edwin states he would "rather see the kids gone," but complains that "my damn wife hassled me so much that I gave in" to having them move South.

Edwin's new civilian job involves extensive shift work and many days away from home. During his subsequent time off–often seven or more days at a stretch–he binge drinks in his basement. While drunk, he quarrels with his children and wife and has become physically assaultive on several occasions. This behavior has resulted in police intervention and frantic calls by Molly to the local mental health center regarding how to handle her husband.

Edwin denies that he has a drinking problem. He states that he drinks only "to get my mind off them damn kids that are running amok. Until that wife of mine started working, the kids weren't any damn problem and I didn't have to drink." He further states that once his wife quits working, he will quit drinking. Molly, however denies that work has anything to do with Edwin's drinking and believes this promise is simply a ploy to "get me stuck at home where he wants me."

Molly has also been in individual-oriented therapy for a number of years for recurrent depression. She frequently calls her therapist after hours and on weekends complaining that she "can't cope" with her husband or job. Occasionally, she abuses prescription drugs such as flurazepam or diazepam. Usually, this follows one of the many quarrels with Edwin.

Since returning home from the military and moving South, Edwin Jr. has dropped out of college and quit three part-time jobs. He states that he is "too depressed" to work or attend school. Both he and his sister Donna use cocaine on a frequent basis. Both have also made periodic calls to the mental health center inquiring about, or occasionally demanding some type of treatment. Most recently, Edwin Jr. called a crisis line and stated that if he did not get into a drug program immediately he would kill himself. He then hung up before he could receive a viable referral.

Donna, the second child, is an extremely attractive young woman who is, by her own description, "a lost soul." Donna dropped out of community college after two semesters, intent on "finding myself . . . you know, travelling or something . . . Doing something exotic." Mostly, however she watches television and helps her mother around the house. Occasionally Donna dances at a topless bar, perhaps to obtain drug money. Other than this occasional stint, she has had no regular employment since high school. Donna rarely dates, stating somewhat realistically that "most men I meet are too scary" to go out with.

Ryan, the youngest child, has recently been suspended from school for getting into fights with other youths. This newest family crisis prompted Molly to call the mental health center for an emergency appointment for her son. Molly quickly terminated Ryan from treatment when she discovered that the therapist wanted to interview the entire family. However, Molly still calls the mental health center for advice when Ryan threatens her or steals some money from other family members.

The therapist was able to work with Donna regarding coaching the family to better handle some of the stressors in their lives. Donna and the therapist met once a week, with each week involving a new "family lesson." In turn, Donna presented these family lessons to her siblings, and later, when they were more compliant, to her parents. These lessons centered around the problems of dysfunctional coping and the need to find more appropriate coping mechanisms. Donna was also able to monitor the family tension and to teach other family members some basic cognitive-behavioral techniques that were useful in controlling some of the helplessness that family members seemed to constantly encounter. Finally, Donna was useful for helping the parents monitor their own substance abuse.

The experience of performing such an important task seemed to boost Donna's self-confidence. She eventually got a job and moved out of the family household. This precipitated another family crisis which eventually was used to help the family accept the need for ongoing treatment.

THE DECISION FOR FUTURE THERAPY

Considerations regarding ongoing and future therapy are often raised with the resistant family and usually can be incorporated into the Behavioral Contract. If the family is in therapy, the considerations are usually brief. The crisis consultant should refer the client family to their therapist as soon as possible with appropriate documentation of any crisis intervention that occurred. At no time should the consultant ever entertain any notions that the therapy may be inappropriate, unless he or she suspects ethical violations on the part of the therapist. This is a most important point. As indicated in Chapter One, resistant families often engage in therapy shopping. Although we have little hesitation in recommending specific treatment modalities to "normal" families, we do not do so in treatment resistant systems. Any complaints regarding the therapist or modality should be politely noted and the patient encouraged to discuss them with the therapist involved.

While this is not an absolute rule, it is a useful guideline we have learned through trial and error. In our less experienced days we would (perhaps intrusively) encourage resistant families in ongoing individual treatment to consider family therapy as an option. Almost invariably, the family would use this suggestion as a reason to terminate its members from individual therapy and would fail to follow through with recommendations for family therapy. The results were generally negative for the functioning of the family system. In fact, data we have collected regarding 56 such recommendations made to resistant families, indicated that 48 resulted in termination of ongoing treatment and a failure to follow through with recommendations for family therapy. Such recommendations with resistant families are hardly effective and also may not be ethical.

We cannot stress enough the importance of the crisis consultant addressing questions regarding ongoing therapy to the ongoing therapist. We used to feel somewhat sheepish about calling therapists after hours for crisis cases, especially regarding crisis-prone families. This is no longer the case. If called on a regular basis, therapists of crisis-prone systems will often take preventive action and communicate a therapeutic plan to potential crisis workers in advance.

If a new appointment for therapy is indicated and the family is agreeable, the worker can either assist the resistant family in making the appointment or entrust the family to do so on their own. If the referral is intra-agency, the former procedure is preferred. This is true despite what we have said about allowing families to make their own mistakes. It is optimal if the family crisis worker can at least temporarily perform case management with the family until a permanent therapist can be found.

We have found we were able to reduce the "no show" rate of families entering new therapy by approximately 30 percent through following two simple guidelines. First, a regular schedule for appointments should be constructed as soon as possible. In the case of an office visit, the therapist should schedule a return session in less than a week, preferably in two to three days. In the instance when telephone or emergency room consultation is required, twenty-four hours is usually the maximal "window" period.

Second, the family should be given limited, but real choices for follow-up appointments. They should be treated as active participants in the initial process (which they are), but restricted in their options for the next appointment. Often a statement such as "I have two openings tomorrow. Which is more convenient?" effectively conveys this message.

TERMINATING THE CRISIS INTERVIEW

Termination of the crisis interview is two-sided. From the consultant's perspective, the establishment of a Behavioral Contract represents the logical point where the family has completed their present task. Before we advocated the routine use of Behavioral Contracts, we used to worry about the proper way to end a session. However, a signed contract is usually the appropriate place to begin to say goodbye to the family, at least for the present. Families almost always sense this and respond accordingly.

The powers of termination also reside with the family. The threat of premature termination, either from the present interview or from further treatment, is often a bargaining chip that resistant families use to gain favored services or avoidance of genuine clinical issues. It usually occurs when specifics are being written into the Behavioral Contract. When the family initiates discussion of termination, the consultant should address it directly. For example, the family may say something like "I don't know if this is helpful, writing all of this down." It may be useful at this point to confront the family's past history of failure and respectfully question whether this pattern will be continued. Then, examples of the usefulness of written treatment agreements with other families can be shared with the vacillating system.

It is rarely useful to bargain with families regarding premature termination from the crisis session or from present or future therapy. Novice therapists frequently plead for resistant families to stay in treatment or to complete a Behavioral Contract. This is a practice the capable consultant does not employ. It is rarely helpful to "break the frame" with a family that threatens to terminate treatment. Families may state they have to quit because of time constraints, location, transportation problems, or a variety of other reasons. The family may ask, for example, to complete the Behavioral Contract at another time, or state they need to end the session because of unforeseen situations, such as a need to return to a babysitter.

Agencies and therapists should be flexible in responding to these needs. However, it is not helpful to add flexibility once the family begins "bargaining" for atypical services, transportation, reduced fees, odd scheduling and the like. Unless there are overriding reasons to the contrary, therapists should avoid extraordinary new measures to secure family compliance and should gently insist that the family continue in completion of the Behavioral Contract.

If the resistant family decides to abruptly terminate a crisis interview it is often helpful to limit their resumption of services for a specified period of time. Naturally, this does not include emergency sessions where there is a danger to self or others. It is also often helpful to specify specific behaviors that must be accomplished prior to re-entry into treatment. We have found it useful, for example, to require family members to attend self-help groups such as Al Anon prior to receiving additional crisis services. This is especially true when the family has a list of reasons for terminating treatment prematurely, none of which are particularly valid in the consultant's opinion.

Sometimes it is useful to have the family review previous treatments prior to offering new crisis intervention or other treatment efforts. During this period, the consultant should be relatively direct regarding past sources of problems related to treatment compliance. A polite, but challenging tone may communicate to the family that the therapist is unsure regarding their motivation for treatment or the likelihood of future compliance.

Regardless of how the crisis interview or any subsequent treatment session ends, the resistant family should terminate any session or treatment effort on a positive but realistic note. The therapist should always be appropriately optimistic regarding the role of therapy in helping the family to meet their needs. On the other hand, it is important to avoid undermining the importance of the family's compliance or the seriousness of their situation.

WHEN ALL ELSE FAILS: REITERATING REALITY TO THE RESISTANT FAMILY

About one quarter of families seen during a crisis will not agree to negotiating a Behavioral Contract. In many cases, the family will simply refuse any treatment recommendations. Or, even more frequently, they may successfully problem solve, yet balk at any specifics that would assist them in translating these gains into manageable behaviors. At this point, the most effective technique is to allow the resistant family to make an informed decision regarding their options. Simply, the consultant states his or her beliefs regarding the family's present and future functioning, outlines a helpful course of action, and then desists in consultation from the system.

We call this process reiterating, since the consultant frequently reiterates what the family should do to improve but is not willing to actually implement at this time.

It is best to keep the content of the reiteration logical (rather than emotional) and succinct. Reiteration works best if it occurs like a respectful broken record. The family may need to hear the same pronouncement repeatedly. Yet they need to hear it optimistically and sincerely. The message should remain encouraging with the emphasis on possible potential change once the family decides to change.

The Family Study below highlights this. Instrumental stress and subsequent crisis with a perceptual "overlay" is involved in this case. The couple are both 30-year-old African-Americans who call to request an emergency appointment. From the history it becomes clear that the family has been in this predicament before, contacted the facility, and failed to follow through on any suggestions that may have been generated from the crisis sessions.

Family Study 8.5. The Bentons

> *Kareem:* We're really in trouble. I mean, I'm so mad, I don't know what to do.
>
> *Consultant:* What seems to be the problem?
>
> *Kareem:* It's my brother. He's had a cocaine problem for a long time. Been arrested more times than I can count. Yolanda and I even paid cash money for his rehab. Up front. Because he let his insurance go. And he was doing good for a while. Going to NA, working . . . and haven't seen him for a year now . . .
>
> *Yolanda:* And what does the son-of-a-bitch do? While we're at work, he breaks into our house and steals everything he can get his ugly hands on. Everything that isn't nailed down.
>
> *Kareem:* Everything. While we're at work. He forges my signature on some checks. Steals the stereo. Empties the savings account. It's just amazing what a person can do in a couple of hours.
>
> *Yolanda:* I had a silver penny my great auntie had from slave times. Gone, probably melted down.

Kareem: We don't know what to do next. If we go to the police, he'll go to jail. For a long time . . . .

Yolanda: If we don't go to the police, forget it. No insurance, nothing.

(At this point the family is engaged in problem solving and agrees to constructing a Behavioral Contract. Twenty minutes are spent generating potential solutions and the couple agrees to involve the police. However, they begin to balk when specifics are discussed.)

Consultant: So we all agree on the need to call the police. Maybe we should put this in writing.

Yolanda. I'd feel better if we had something in writing . . .

Kareem: No! So what are they gonna do? They'll think, this is just another nigger running some scam. I don't want to even call the police. They won't believe me. And then they'll be questioning me at work. They don't understand that kind of shit where I work. Okay, like I work around a lot of white folks. The only cop they've seen is in the movies or at a parking meter. Man, I'm the manager with 20 people under me. I'm making good money. They'll fire me up front for suspicion. I'm ruined.

Yolanda (to Kareem): You have to call the police.

Kareem: I mean, we don't want to send him to jail for slipping up, but I mean . . . I feel its him against me. One more time.

Yolanda: You mean it's him against your children. We won't even be able to pay the mortgage this month.

Kareem: (Very devastated) If they fire me for this kind of shit we can't pay the mortgage.

Consultant: From what I recall, you all have gone through this several times–I mean the cycle of not knowing what to do.

Kareem: Yeah, that's right.

Consultant: I don't want to advise you what to do. But you know, by not doing something–and that's pretty much been your pattern by not doing something, you really are just making sure that your brother has his way.

Yolanda: That's what I've been saying!

Kareem. It won't help. Calling the police won't help him.

Consultant: Maybe not. But I am struck by the fact that you keep trying to solve his problems–the problems he causes–by not doing anything. It won't work. It's like beating your head against the wall.

Yolanda: It's hopeless. I know what you are getting at.

Consultant: I understand how you feel. But it's only hopeless if you don't try. As long as you don't, well, the problem will keep recurring.

Kareem: You sure?

Consultant: Pretty much, yeah. It will get worse.

In this instance, reiteration was successful. The family agreed to call the police about the brother. Later they pursued additional therapy for themselves.

Reiteration occasionally involves communicating to the family the likelihood they will be forced into some type of ongoing treatment. Usually, this occurs when there is court supervision and the therapist has been charged with the responsibility of communicating the family's progress to a probation officer. Such relationships are fraught with difficulties, not the least being that trust is typically compromised by this arrangement. As we have stated throughout this volume, it is our philosophy to avoid forcing the family into ongoing treatment, inasmuch as forced treatment does not seem to be effective. It is also counterproductive inasmuch as it tends to further convince the family that treatment is ineffective and imposed by someone outside of the family system.

Experience with resistant systems has encouraged us to avoid mandated treatment. For example, we no longer believe that forced compliance for families of schizophrenics or personality disorders is helpful. Forced family treatment for depressive disorders is rarely helpful, except in the cases of adolescent depression. We are only moderately enthusiastic about forced family treatment of domestic violence, and increasingly prefer to work with abusers and victims separately until they have sufficient desire to change their behaviors, or make use of alternate options.

Forced treatment compliance is ethically mandated where a resistant system coexists with the likelihood of exploitation on the part of system members. These cases include child abuse and incest, but may also include cases where a member of the client family is cognitively impaired or brain damaged. Each of these instances will be discussed in following chapters.

BEYOND THE CRISIS SESSION: WHAT TO DO WITH THE RESISTANT FAMILY AFTER ADEPT

The focus of this book has been on actions that the therapist/consultant can perform in one to three sessions (or occasionally more) to treat extremely resistant family systems. Our interventions have been designed to weaken and circumvent resistance before it becomes problematic. After negotiating all of the steps in the ADEPT model, there are four possible outcomes that the worker and the family may experience

In the most felicitous situation, the family may be "cured." We use this term loosely, since all systems have a degree of instability. The concept of cure is derived largely from the linear model of pathology and implies a single entity is "broken" and can be fixed. This is seldom a useful concept in working with resistant families. But what *can* happen is that the presenting crisis may have challenged the family to abruptly and positively change. The therapist/consultant may then have been able to supplant enough functional homeostatic mechanisms into the system that the family will emerge with a different and superior level of self-organization. The following family study illustrates this potentiality.

Family Study 8.6. The Barnes

Linda and Donald Barnes became involved in couples' treatment after Don's psychoanalyst suggested marital therapy.

The couple had resisted the analyst's suggestion for several months, despite their deteriorating marriage. Linda, a mid-level executive for an oil company, had a tendency towards severe binge drinking. Don was a director of nursing at a large hospital who believed his professional skills gave him the ability to treat his wife without outside help. Don finally called a family therapist while in crisis. The day before Linda had become inappropriately drunk at a neighbor's house during a social event and Don called to say he had enough.

During the crisis session it became apparent that the use of alcohol was the principal mechanism by which Linda felt she could be assertive regarding her sexual and emotional needs. A problem-solving session generated other ways in which she could more functionally express her desires to her husband. Following implementation of these solutions through a Behavioral Contract, Linda stopped drinking almost immediately. Several months later the couple was seen for follow-up. They reported being basically happy, arguing much less, and having better and more caring sex.

"Cures" of this type do not happen too frequently. They do occur occasionally, even in surprisingly severe cases. However, in situations where there is a rapid symptom reduction in a previously resistant family, we recommend periodic booster sessions or monitoring to ensure that systemic changes are maintained. Sessions should be scheduled for once a month or so until the family and the therapist/consultant are reasonably confident that the problem has been resolved. At that point the therapist/consultant needs to reiterate an "open door policy" regarding relapse. The family should be inoculated to the fact that they may again slip into their former behavior patterns. There should be no stigma about receiving further treatment if necessary.

A more common outcome in our crisis intervention/consultation protocol is that the resistant family is persuaded that they need additional help. This help may not necessarily be from a professional. It could include self-help, religious involvement, or additional family supports. The appropriateness of the referral depends both upon the family's presenting problem and their level of resistance. The Family Study below illustrates this type of outcome.

Family Study 8.7. The Ellinsky Family

Jerry and Sylvia Ellinsky were a late middle-aged couple with three college-age children living far from home. The couple, both professors, fought constantly and were miserable. Jerry drank heavily, often in response to quarrels at home about his lack of sexual interest. Sylvia rather openly flaunted an extramarital affair with a neighbor. The couple had attempted separation, but were even more miserable, partially because they were excessively dependent upon each other and very disagreeable toward most other people. They also did not want to divorce because of religious reasons.

Both Jerry and Sylvia had tried a variety of therapies, with seemingly no benefit. The couple called a family therapist specializing in working with resistant families only after Jerry was arrested for drunk driving.

During the first crisis session Jerry steadfastly denied that he had a drinking problem. The therapist challenged him to prove it by instructing him to take only one drink a day for the next month. This proved impossible for even two days and Jerry returned to the next session admitting that he needed alcohol treatment.

In the meantime, Sylvia and Jerry were able to problem solve ways to manage a trial separation. During the separation, Jerry received outpatient substance abuse therapy. Sylvia eventually ended her affair. The couple ultimately reunited and continued ongoing marital therapy. Jerry's libido gradually improved with the cessation of drinking and enhanced communications with his wife.

There are no hard rules for what type of therapy is appropriate for families making the transition from crisis-oriented interventions described in this volume to longer-term modalities. Discrete problems need to be addressed with treatment specific modalities. For example, if a major problem in the system concerns difficulties with family hierarchies, then a structural approach might be indicated. If communications deficits are pronounced, then behavioral family interventions might be warranted. Closed systems may need more humanistic interventions. Problems with triangling may require a more Bowenian approach, while excessive "baggage" with family members' parents and siblings suggests analytic family interventions.

Obviously, no one therapist can develop expertise in all of these techniques. If we had only one method to master for resistant families being transitioned to a more permanent treatment we would choose the therapeutic procedures of L'Abate (1986). L'Abate's framework offers an excellent theory-based series of techniques that cover a variety of issues applicable to resistant Systems. L'Abate is a defender of both eclecticism and empiricism, and of careful assessment of the system before interventions are negotiated. His work, a hallmark of scholarship, also highlights two major themes encountered in resistant families: intimacy and termination. Furthermore, he provides excellent structured exercises, based on his general emphasis on therapeutic writing, that we have found extremely useful with resistant systems. Finally, he furnishes a methodology for an important variable in family therapy, namely outcome research.

The third possible outcome of families treated by our method is probably the most common, especially for resistant systems. Family tension is reduced somewhat and the crisis gradually abates. However, the family does not consent to additional treatment, or worse, consents and fails to follow through. Yet the family has learned a few more coping skills, so that they are perhaps a bit less crisis-prone. They may have also learned less reliance on dysfunctional coping mechanisms, so that their prospects for longer term functioning are improved.

From a research standpoint, these families are the most interesting to us. They often continue to make changes long after the cessation of the therapy. These families may make initial contact and then terminate quickly. Two or three years later the therapist quite unexpectedly hears from them. They report that their lives have been changed and attribute the difference to the therapist's interventions. The therapist thinks back in disbelief, hardly able to remember the family at all. Possibly, these families are the most gratifying of all.

Sometimes change within these systems follows an extremely minimal intervention which may not sustain results for months or years. One of the authors recently received a letter from a family that was seen in crisis eight years ago. The family never returned for a second session. By all conventional accounts they were a clear treatment failure. However, their letter reported numerous positive changes, occurring slowly and over a number of years. These changes were attributed to a single ninety-minute session, conducted entirely by telephone in the middle of the night.

Finally, there is the all too common family system that doesn't seem to benefit from our interventions whatsoever. They have resisted therapy in the past and will continue to do so in the future. No noticeable inroads have been made during this most recent cycle of crisis and termination. When families such as these are seen again, and they will be, the therapist/consultant must not loose faith in the possibility that they can eventually change. In the meantime, he or she must be content with the knowledge that the seeds of change may have been planted and that no harm has been done.

Chapter Nine

When the Resistant Family
Is Incestuous

Data from McCown and Johnson (1991) suggest that as many as 10 percent of high risk families have a history of incest for one or more members. Furthermore, perhaps one in twenty-five cases of family-oriented crisis intervention may involve a precipitating problem directly or indirectly related to incest. When families are actively involved in perpetrating incest, many of the brief, problem-oriented techniques advocated in this volume are inappropriate. For example, we cannot let the resistant family continue its dysfunctional behavior when incest or other forms of child abuse is involved, regardless of our general belief that systems in crisis need to assume responsibility for their own actions and behavioral change. Incest or child abuse demands alternative treatment interventions, some of which the family-oriented crisis therapist is ill-prepared or disinclined to advocate. Often these include individual therapy with mandated therapeutic compliance, techniques that are seldom useful for other resistant family difficulties.

The focus of this chapter is to provide guidelines for conducting family therapy with treatment resistant families where intrafamilial sexual abuse has occurred. Although much of this chapter is also applicable to cases of physical abuse where there is no concurrent sexual exploitation, we focus primarily on the latter problem because of its significance with resistant families. We being with a discussion of the controversy surrounding family therapy with incestuous families and a statement of general principles. After a brief outline of the issues involved in interacting with other agencies, an assessment model is presented. The chapter concludes with an inte-

grated summary regarding family therapy and other treatment modalities and a discussion of therapeutic goals.

GENERAL PRINCIPLES

The discussion of incest is capable of arousing powerful emotional reactions, and the idea of conducting family therapy with
incestuous families has provoked heated debate (e.g., Carter et al.,
1986). Opposition to family therapy in cases of incest is due in part
to the conflict between the victim-perpetrator model and the family
systems model (Trepper & Barrett, 1986a). The "victim-perpetrator
model" is a linear model in which incest is viewed as the aggressive
act of a pathological or deviant adult perpetrator against an innocent
or uninvolved victim (Trepper & Barrett, 1986a). Workers in child
protective services and also many crisis therapists typically follow
this model and emphasize victim advocacy, external control of incestuous families, and an individual approach to treatment (Larson
& Maddock, 1986). Trepper and Barrett (1986a) assert the model is
popular because (1) there is obvious truth to a model that recognizes
the greater capacity of the adult perpetrator; (2) the model is simple–it is linear, directional, and intuitive; and (3) the model allows
us to keep a certain psychological distance from the behavior in
question.

The second model, family systems, views incestuous or other
abusive activities as the product of a problematic family system
rather than as the cause, and sees all family members as sharing in
its development (Trepper & Barrett, 1986a). Systems-oriented therapists believe that a linear assignment of blame or responsibility is
naive in its understanding of circular and interactional forces within
the family which become expressed in symptomatic behavior (Grunebaum, 1987).

Many feminists criticize the systems perspective regarding incest
and other forms of child abuse (Carter et al., 1986; Grunebaum,
1987). Feminist therapists who are not family therapists maintain
that current models of family therapy ignore the issue of personal
accountability for the incestuous act, are insensitive to the ways in
which the problem of incest reflects unequal power relations within

the social and economic structure at large, and disregard inequalities pertaining to relative responsibilities of men and women as parents (Grunebaum, 1987). Conte (1986) asserts that traditional family therapists tend to support established sex-role stereotyped power distributions in families in spite of the fact that fundamental alterations in parental power are necessary when such power has been used to coerce or manipulate a child into a sexual relationship (Conte, 1986).

Another objection to family therapy in cases of incest, and, to a lesser extent, other forms of abuse, springs from concern that family therapy will allow for further victimization of the child. This may be especially true for the resistant family. Concern for the revictimization of the child must be the first priority, but it is naive to think that a victim-perpetrator approach automatically prevents revictimization. This approach ignores the trauma that is caused by taking the child away from parents or by removing the offending parent (Pardeck, 1989; Pernett & Urwitz, 1990; Trepper & Barrett, 1986a). Often the child has a deep loyalty to the offending parent and will assume self-blame regarding the event (Grunebaum, 1987). Similarly, family members, both parents and siblings, frequently blame the victim for the crisis that follows the disclosure and reject the child rather than face the crisis directly (Giaretto, 1989; Grunebaum, 1987). Foster or adoptive placements, if they can be found, do not necessarily represent salvation for a child, and legal procedures themselves can serve to victimize the child. As energy is focused on building a criminal case, the child can be put through many explicit interviews by different authorities, and may even be asked to testify against his/her parent in court. The child may experience guilt regarding his/her role in sending a parent to prison (Cornille, 1989). Another possible negative consequence of the victim-perpetrator approach is that if agencies are unable to terminate parental rights, the family may be reunited without the potential benefits of therapy.

The approach taken here attempts to recognize the validity of all of the above perspectives; it takes the position that family therapy–but generally not brief, crisis-oriented interventions–may be a useful therapeutic approach with some resistant families in some cases of intrafamilial sexual abuse. Both the victim-perpetrator model and the family systems model are probably simplistic. It is likely the etiology of incest is far more complex and includes sociocultural, family, individual personality, family of origin, and situational factors (Trepper & Sprenkle, 1989). This chapter advocates the use of the Multiple Systems Perspective of Trepper & Barrett (1986a) as an organizing framework in approaching intrafamilial sexual abuse, especially regarding resistant systems.

It is hoped the following basic principles will answer some of the above mentioned objections to family therapy in incest cases:

1. Child protection must be the first priority of all therapists. This is especially true for emergency workers.
2. Sexual contact between an adult and a child is always the responsibility of the adult. Non-offending adults in the family should also be held accountable for their actions or lack of action. This does not preclude concern for these adults. It does, however, state that the responsibilities to the child come before those to the rest of the family.
3. Brief, problem-focused therapy, often helpful for resistant families, is rarely appropriate for cases of incest or other forms of sexual abuse. Incestual families cannot be allowed the "luxury to fail," as other families are. The consequences are simply too great.
4. The family approach is not advocated in all cases of intrafamilial sexual abuse, and should generally be conducted in conjunction with other treatment modalities (e.g., individuals, groups, and dyads).

INITIAL INTERVENTION

The point at which the incest has been discovered will have a major impact on the way therapy proceeds. If the therapist is involved with the family at the point of discovery of the incest, the first stage is usually one of prevention of victimization. While a Behavioral Contract may be of value during this phase, this is generally accomplished by reporting the abuse to child protective services or law enforcement agencies. In most states such reporting is required by law.

More often, initial contact with the incestuous family occurs when one or more family members seek mental health consultation or crisis intervention as new clients. One or more individuals within the family system may be acutely suicidal. The appropriate interventions for families in this stage are the typical family crisis intervention techniques discussed earlier. However, invariably, therapists will have to assume more of a direct, ego-involved role, rather than a more removed, consultant stance. This is because the damage that incest typically wrecks in families often effectively impairs their ability to adequately problem solve for their members. Behavioral Contracts negotiated with such families usually have to be extraordinarily specific and conservative, since such families are often "concrete" regarding their incest-related behaviors.

One of the first decisions that needs to be made once the sexual abuse is discovered is whether the abusing parent will be removed from the home, the child will be removed from the home, both the abusing parent and child will be removed from the home, or whether both will remain in the home. Some of the possible adverse consequences of breaking up the family were noted earlier. Very likely this decision will be out of the hands of the therapist and made by the local protective service agency and law enforcement personnel. Therapists may play a role in the investigation, however, and be asked for recommendations. Assessment during the investigation phase should focus on the history of harm that has been caused and the family's ability to maintain enough control over its actions to protect family members from harm (Cornille, 1989), as well as their likelihood of remaining in treatment. Specific assessment recommendations are made below. The decision that is made regarding separation of family members will exert a dramatic impact on the course of treatment.

Coordination of efforts with other agencies is mandatory in any incest case and even more important with the resistant family. Such coordination should be a part of the treatment plan. Many different people become involved with a child abuse case once it is reported. These may include police, protective service/social service workers, district attorneys, public defenders, probation officers, and treatment professionals. The number of different people working on the case can make it confusing even for experienced professionals, let alone for the family that has been assigned a different social worker by each system (Pernett & Urwitz, 1990). In addition to the problems of sheer numbers of professionals, each group or "system" has a different perspective on the case. When the various systems do not respond sensitively, they are less likely to gain the trust of the parties involved. Satisfactory resolution of the matter then becomes improbable, and revictimization of the child is likely.

The therapist must exercise care to ensure that he or she does not get encumbered in the myth that systems outside the family are dangerous to and designed to destroy the family. This sentiment is especially common in treatment resistant families. Therapists must try to understand the perspectives of other systems, and they should keep in mind that their goals are the same–to protect the child and keep abuse from recurring. Current uncoordinated responses are preventing those goals from being met and are driving cases of abuse underground (Giaretto, 1989; Pernett & Urwitz, 1990). Through purposeful cooperation with social agencies, the therapist can ensure that the necessary level of protection for the child is maintained throughout therapy (Cornille, 1989). Under these circumstances, the level of responsibility that the family and individual family members are capable of managing should grow with time and nurturance (Cornille, 1989).

Given the degree of emotionality typically surrounding incestuous behavior, there is a great likelihood that the therapist's values and sentiment concerning the families and their behavior will interfere with objective analysis (Carr, 1989; Trepper and Barrett, 1986a). This is even more common when the family system attempts to thwart intervention or is nonplussed regarding the sexual abuse that has occurred, as resistant families frequently are. One concern is the level of anger the therapist may feel toward the perpetrator and perhaps toward other members of the family. Emergency workers, in particular, often seem to have extraordinary difficulty with incestuous families, and this anger may cloud their clinical judgment. Carr (1989) describes five such reactions, including fantasies of rescuing the child from the family; rescuing the mother and child and persecuting the father; rescuing the parents from a hostile social environment and a punitive child protection system; rescuing the father (rare); and persecuting the family. Although these feelings may be understandable, they can substantially interfere with accurate assessment and treatment. The therapist needs to be aware of his/her own values and any countertransference reactions, and cognizant of the manner in which these reactions may bias clinical decision making. To assist in maintaining some level of objectivity, Barrett, Sykes and Byrnes (1986) recommend co-therapy and ongoing supervision. At this point it is necessary to indicate that the writers refer to the perpetrator as the father because the majority of incestuous relationships involve the father or another male figure in the family.

Dimensions of Assessment

There has been a movement away from the assumption that there is one profile for families in which incest occurs; hence, a variety of descriptions of individual family members, family dynamics, and environmental determinants are found in the literature (Trepper & Barrett, 1986a). Unfortunately, these descriptions are usually not based upon empirical findings, but rather on clinical observations of small samples (Trepper & Barrett, 1986a). These varied descriptions probably result in part from the diversity of incestuous families, and should inform the clinician that the characteristics of sexually abusive families cannot be assumed a priori. Rather, they must be identified through clinical assessment (Conte, 1986), beginning with the initial family session.

A thorough assessment of the family will enable the clinician to develop a sensible intervention strategy tailored to the needs of that particular family. An error that crisis-oriented therapists sometimes make with incestual families is in assuming that initial and crisis-oriented assessments such as those advocated in this volume are sufficient to engage in treatment planning and service delivery. Instead, we advocate several additional areas of assessment suggested by current literature.

Nature of the Abuse

An examination of the nature of the abuse provides a good starting point. Some of the critical variables which should ideally emerge from the initial investigation are: the age of the child at the time of abuse, the level of physical aggression involved, and the extent of abuse. The extent of the sexual abuse can be assessed along the dimensions of duration, frequency, and intrusiveness (Faller, 1988). On a continuum from least to most, intrusiveness consists of (1) noncontact sexual abuse (inappropriate sexual statements to the child, exposure, voyeurism); (2) sexual contact (fondling, mutual masturbation, frottage); (3) oral sex (sucking of breasts, cunnilingus, fellatio); and (4) penetration (anal, genital) (Faller, 1988). Other aspects of the sexual abuse concern whether pictures are taken, whether the perpetrator allows or forces others to engage in sex with the child, how many victims there are, and whether victims are both intrafamilial and extrafamilial (Faller, 1988).

The Multiple Systems Perspective

In addition to the nature of the abuse, the clinician should examine those factors contributing to the abuse. Trepper and Barrett (1986b) have posited a diathesis/stress model for the development of intrafamilial sexual abuse that provides a useful framework to guide assessment. Their "Multiple Systems Perspective" is an eco-systemic model that views incest as resulting from a number of factors related to a variety of systems (Trepper & Sprenkle, 1989). The vulnerability factors that they propose include (1) family of origin; (2) personality characteristics of family members; (3) family system factors; and (4) socio-environmental factors. The actual occurrence of incest, however, depends on a precipitating stressful event and the absence of functional coping mechanisms. The underlying premise of their model is exactly the same as that of family crisis vulnerability discussed earlier; there is no singular cause of intrafamily sexual abuse. Instead, all families are endowed with a degree of vulnerability, based upon individual, family, and environmental factors, which may be expressed as incest if a precipitating event takes place and the family's coping skills are low. Trepper and Barrett (1986b) note that the goal of clinical assessment is to obtain information regarding which factors in their model are present that made the family particularly vulnerable, what precipitants were involved, and where the family's coping mechanisms are lacking. A treatment plan can then be developed with goals to reduce vulnerability, decrease possible precipitants, and increase family coping skills (Trepper & Barrett, 1986b).

FAMILY SYSTEM FACTORS

Trepper and Barrett (1986b) identify three levels of systemic functioning which may contribute to a family's vulnerability: family structure, family style, and communication patterns.

Family structure refers to the organization of a family with regard to roles, hierarchies, rules, and power (Minuchin, 1974). Dysfunctional family structure has often been mentioned in the literature as a contributor to the occurrence of incest. Trepper and Barrett (1986b) make use of Olson's Circumplex Model which looks at family structure along the dimensions of adaptability and cohesion. Cohesion refers to the level of emotional connectedness between family members and ranges from enmeshed to disengaged. Adaptability refers to capacity for change and ranges from chaotic to rigid. On the Circumplex, most of these families typically fall in the extreme ranges (Trepper & Barrett, 1986b; Trepper & Sprenkle, 1989). The most common two-dimensional patterns among their population of incestuous families are rigid-enmeshed and chaotic-enmeshed. The combination of an overly strict adherence to rules and the secretiveness which follows, combined with personal over-involvement with each other's emotional lives and concomitant social isolation, renders the rigid-enmeshed family particularly vulnerable to incest (Trepper & Sprenkle, 1989). Trepper & Sprenkle (1989) recommend the use of FACES III and the Clinical Rating Scales for assessing family structure, both of which are based on the Circumplex Model. It is important to realize that these instruments should not be used during a crisis situation, inasmuch as reliability is apt to be reduced, especially for resistant families.

A family structure classification more specific to intrafamily sexual abuse is described by Trepper and Barrett (1986b). They describe the structures believed to be vulnerable to incest as father executive, mother executive, third generation, and chaotic. In the "father executive" family, the father is the executive, and the daughter has reversed roles with the mother, who is either emotionally or physically absent from the family. In "mother executive" families, the mother is the sole executive, and the father functions like one of the children. Trepper and Barrett (1986b) describe families where the mother functions like a grandmother as "third generation." The mother parents the father who fluctuates between being a parent and a sibling to his children. The "chaotic family" is one in which there is no executive subsystem. The parents and children function on the same level with regard to their formal roles, and no one enforces rules or boundaries.

Larson and Maddock (1986) also propose that boundary disturbances between the adult and child generations and between family members contribute to incest. They describe boundaries between adult and child generations as "blurred." Children become "parentified" and respond in a way that is adaptive in the short-run, while promoting in the long-run a grandiose belief that they are capable of meeting any and all emotional needs of other people, even at their own expense. Personal boundaries become diffuse, and interaction produces symbiotic relationship patterns in which each member feels that his/her survival is dependent on the emotional and psychosocial status of the other members. Differentiation of self, involving independent thought, feeling, desire, and behavior by family members, is threatening to the structure of the incestuous family system. Differentness or uniqueness is experienced as distance, and individuality is viewed as alienation and disloyalty. Control becomes a critical factor in family structure, and members who threaten the system through autonomous behavior can become the targets of scapegoating and escalating abuse (Larson and Maddock, 1986). It should be acknowledged that it is difficult, if not impossible, to determine whether disturbed family structure is the cause or the result of incest (Conte, 1986).

Family style is defined by Trepper & Barrett (1986b) as the pervasive and enduring patterns of interaction a family displays. These patterns are reflected in the particular meaning and function of the incestuous behavior in a given system. Larson and Maddock (1986) state that sexual involvement with children serves one of four basic functions: (1) affectional process; (2) erotic process;

(3) aggression process; and (4) process of expressing rage. All of these processes serve to restore homeostasis to the stressed family unit, and therefore possess some degree of functionality for the family system. The therapist must attempt to understand the function of the abuse for the perpetrator and the family. In addition, he or she must address family myths, secrets, themes, and belief systems. These common cognitive sets may function as mediators for sexual abuse, either eliciting certain kinds of behavior, providing a rationalization for other kinds of behavior, or preventing or suppressing alternative behaviors (Conte, 1986).

The therapist should examine how each family member responded to the disclosure of the abuse. He or she may want to assess the level of empathy that parents have for their children as well as the level of loyalty the children feel toward their parents. It is important to understand the meaning of the abuse for the victim. The therapist must be concerned with how a sense of worth is being validated or disconfirmed for members of the family, especially the children (Grunebaum, 1987).

Family communication in sexually abusive families commonly reflects conflict avoidance, secretiveness, hostility, and double-binding communication (Trepper & Barrett, 1986b). Incestuous clients are frequently inept at communicating their feelings, needs, and points of view. Thus, their problem-solving abilities are often inadequate and superficial within their marital and family systems (Taylor, 1986).

Unfortunately, these family deficits are common among most resistant families and are not in themselves pathognomonic of incest. Often, ongoing therapy with such families will involve extra session crisis intervention regarding these basic issues. The therapeutic task is to teach the incestuous client communicate directly and clearly and how to use that communication to solve problems both within and outside the family system (Taylor, 1986).

INDIVIDUAL FACTORS

A thorough assessment of the individual characteristics of the various family members should be conducted outside of the basic crisis intervention session provided for resistant families. Some commentators have suggested specific areas that they consider important. For example, Faller (1988) states there are certain characteristics of maternal and paternal caretakers that are crucial to intervention decisions. Important characteristics for fathers are: (1) overall functioning; (2) level of moral functioning; and (3) the extent of the sexual abuse. General functioning can be assessed from the perpetrator's education, work history, mental health, substance use, functioning in the community, criminal activity, behavior as a spouse, and relationship with his children. Moral functioning should be evaluated with particular attention to remorse or guilt regarding the sexual abuse. Faller asserts the prospects of change sufficient for adequate parental functioning are remote in the individual who has engaged in extensive sexual abuse, has few areas of appropriate functioning, and little or no guilt about the sexual abuse. In contrast, if he has many areas of appropriate functioning, extensive guilt regarding the sexual abuse, and has engaged in minimal sexual behavior, the prospects for rehabilitation are much better. Trepper and Barrett (1986b) also examine the father's degree of sociopathic characteristics, level of dominance and aggressiveness, adequacy of sexual functioning, and need for love and adoration.

For mothers, Faller (1988) states the crucial characteristics to be: (1) level of her dependency, particularly upon the perpetrator; (2) degree to which she loves and is nurturing of the victim (and other children); and (3) extent to which she was protective when she discovered the sexual abuse. The three maternal factors, taken together, are predictive of the change potential of the mother. Mothers who are dependent, who blame or are hostile toward the victim, and who are unprotective of their children are not likely to change sufficiently to become adequate parents. In contrast, the mother who is independent, nurturing, and protective will be better able to make necessary changes and may be able to assist the perpetrator in changing. Trepper and Barrett (1986b) also examine the mother's degree of passivity, dependence, self-esteem, and sexual functioning.

Distortions of sexuality on the part of the family and individual family members must be addressed and are a commonly encountered problem when the resistant family is incestuous. Some possible problems related to sexuality are outlined in Larson and Maddock (1986) and include lack of respect for personal privacy, both physical and emotional; lack of knowledge about sex, lack of an effective communication system regarding sex, including paucity of feelings expressed and attitude distortion; and lack of an overall sexual value system to transmit from one generation to the next. Other identified difficulties entail a paucity of information exchange regarding sex-related beliefs, attitudes, and values; lack of a satisfactory and mutually meaningful erotic relationship in the marital dyad, including loss of expressiveness, reduced affection exchange, and little capacity for negotiation of sexual interest; poor body/self-image, and a general shame-based, negative view of sex and the body. Along similar lines, Taylor (1986) states that sexual uncertainty, sexual insecurity, and lack of sexual knowledge are all prevalent among incestuous clients and contribute directly to the incestuous behavior.

FAMILY OF ORIGIN FACTORS

Many writers assert that parents in incestuous families were very often victims of abuse themselves. It is therefore important to assess the parents' past history of abuse, including the degree of emotional deprivation or neglect they may have experienced as children (Trepper & Barrett, 1986b).

Unfortunately, treatment resistant families will also be highly secretive regarding these issues. Probing by the therapist with such families may even institute future crises. Barker (1990) notes that many emergency room visits are precipitated by the uncovering of past sexual traumas. In our experience, this holds equally true for the perpetrator as well as the victim. In some cases the crisis response from uncovered memories in family therapy will be so profound that psychiatric hospitalization must be considered.

SOCIO-ENVIRONMENTAL FACTORS

Social isolation is often considered a key factor in both the development of incestuous behavior and in the intensification of the molestation over time (Taylor, 1986). Larson and Maddock (1986) state that incestuous families protect their sexual secret by constructing barriers between the family system and its social environment. Our anecdotal accounts suggest that incestuous families are grossly deficient in social supports, especially from those outside of the family. The tolerance toward incestuous behavior in the community in which the family lives, as well as the general cultural acceptance of male dominance, may also contribute to the occurrence of incest.

PRECIPITATING EVENTS

Trepper and Barrett (1986b) note that precipitating events may include: (1) substance abuse; (2) mother's absence from home; or (3) major acute stress. They emphasize that these are never "causes" of incest. Taylor (1986) states that feelings of abandonment or a major loss of self-esteem experienced by the perpetrator which results from job loss, health problems, career setbacks, financial problems, marital discord, or emotional or physical distancing by the adult female can contribute to incestuous behavior.

The therapist who evaluates a client from an incestuous system may be called upon to help the client family manage acute present stressors so the event is not repeated. Often, this will involve more ego-lending than usual, with the therapist performing an exaggerated amount of problem solving for the family. As long as anyone in the family system is at risk, it is our sentiment that the therapist must remain active and cannot let the system decide when and how to change. Some therapists may recoil from this suggestion, feeling this may serve to "infantilize" the family or increase dependency of the family on the therapist. Although we recognize these concerns, we believe that the dangers of incest outweigh those from increasing the system's dependency on an outside agent.

COPING MECHANISMS

As we have indicated throughout the volume, the clinician should assess the family's styles for coping in an effort to discover adaptive as well as maladaptive mechanisms. Trepper and Barrett (1986b) suggest the Family Strengths and Family Coping Strategies Inventories which provide information on dimensions such as problem solving abilities, availability of extended family, ability to recognize and utilize social networks, and degree of religious beliefs are useful assessment tools. Again, we do not advocate this data be obtained during crises, as it is apt to be somewhat unreliable. On the other hand, the assessments of coping suggested in this volume seem relatively impervious to distortion from a crisis situation and may be particularly helpful for the incestuous and resistant family.

DIMENSIONS OF INTERVENTION

Unfortunately, there is little guidance available to the mental health professional attempting to determine the potential of different types of sexually abusive families to benefit from treatment, nor is there much guidance on case management strategies (Faller, 1988). There is an absence of empirical data demonstrating the relative efficacy of particular theoretical orientations or demonstrating one particular unit of treatment (such as individual, marital couple, or whole family) as specifically indicated in the treatment of child sexual abuse (Kolko, 1987). Although some optimistic treatment outcomes have been reported by multidisciplinary programs with family involvement, there is little in the way of supporting data (Kolko, 1987).

Most authors suggest the integration of treatment modalities including both individual-focused and family-focused approaches. These may include individual sessions with the nonabusing parent as well as with the offender and child. Other authors suggest the addition of group sessions, marital sessions, mother-daughter sessions, father-daughter sessions, sibling sessions, or sessions with the parents' families of origin. The sequence of treatment strategies has been found to be highly variable across programs, and only a few programs provide clear guidelines regarding the order in which therapy procedures are introduced or an underlying conceptual orientation (Kolko, 1987). However, individual therapy is generally offered first. One comprehensive multi-disciplinary team approach which has been extensively described in the literature is the Child Sexual Abuse Treatment Program (CSATP) of Santa Clara County, California (1989). In this program, treatment activities are conducted in the following sequence: (1) individual counselling for the child, mother, and father; (2) mother-daughter counselling; (3) marital therapy; (4) father-daughter counselling; (5) family therapy; and (6) group therapy (Kolko, 1987).

Therapists should probably see the child and each parent individually until they reach a point where they are ready for family sessions (Pardeck, 1989). Some families, especially those who are treatment resistant, may never reach that point. One reason individual sessions with the child are necessary is to ensure that the child victim will report incidents of sexual abuse that may occur during the course of treatment. Subsequent crisis intervention of incestuous families should always include a substantial individual component. This is one of the few situations where we advocate individual-oriented crisis intervention as a standard of care.

The following recommendations are drawn from family commentators from a variety of theoretical perspectives, including humanistic (Giaretto, 1982), contextual (Grunebaum, 1987), and a combination of structural, strategic and systemic (Trepper & Barrett, 1986b; Trepper & Sprenkle, 1989).

Targets of Intervention

As indicated in the Assessment section, incest families can vary on a number of different dimensions, and the targets of intervention are essentially the same as the targets for assessment: family factors, family of origin factors, individual factors, socio-environmental factors, precipitating events, and coping skills.

Accountability

One of the first treatment problems likely to be encountered is denial, both by the child and the abusing parent. Denial and related defense mechanisms, used consistently over time, impair feedback processes within the family and distort members' perceptions of outside reality (Larson & Maddock, 1986). Believing they must continue certain behaviors to survive, family members remain stuck in their destructive victim/victimizer patterns, thereby increasing their feelings of shame and powerlessness. In turn, the feelings promote further isolation and perceptual distortion. Due to the protective nature of denial, family members are usually thrown into a crisis when the incest secret is revealed to the outside world and/or is openly confronted within the family for the first time (Larson & Maddock, 1986). While this pattern is typical of almost all resistant systems, it is most pronounced with incestuous systems.

There are differences of opinion regarding the therapeutic necessity of having the offender take responsibility for his incestuous behavior, but the majority of therapists seem to require such acceptance of responsibility. Cornille (1989) states the perpetrator must recognize that final responsibility for the sexual act is exclusively his, and cannot be abdicated to the wife, victim, or the perpetrator's childhood experiences. The mother must be willing to act in a protective manner towards her children, including supporting the victim's decision to ask for help (Cornille, 1989).

Grunebaum (1987) asserts that each individual may be differentially addressed in terms of his or her constructive and destructive "contributions to the system." Thus, the father's responsibility for engaging in sexual relations with his daughter, for example, can be distinguished from the mother's responsibility to take care of and protect her daughter. Responsibility can be viewed within the context of relative influence in the larger society and within the family—those who have the most power have the greatest responsibility not to abuse it (Grunebaum, 1987). However, while the offender should be held accountable, condemnation and scapegoating should never occur. The perpetrator must be helped to regain the respect and trust of his family; this is in the long-term interest of all the children (Grunebaum, 1987). For example, the "apology session" is described by Trepper (1986) as a useful early stage intervention to quickly and dramatically institute change in the sexually abusive family by having the parents each accept their share of responsibility for the abuse. Trepper says that a number of elements are crucial to the success of the apology session: (1) each parent must be genuinely sorry for his or her portion of responsibility and must genuinely not want the abuse to occur again; (2) the parents must demonstrate cohesiveness in giving children the message that the problem is their responsibility; and (3) the session should remain focused on the apology, the responsibility of each family member to make things better, and the promise of better things to come. The apology session should also help to alleviate the guilt feelings of the abused child (Barrett, Sykes, & Byrnes, 1986). Children may continue to feel angry with their parents, and may not even feel safe with them, but they should allow their parents the chance to make their family better (Trepper, 1986).

Care needs to be taken in implementing an apology session when the family system is treatment resistant. The emotions such a session unleashes may require extensive subsequent treatment to defuse. Therapists who arrange an apology session for a family that will shortly drop out of treatment probably do far more harm than good. Therefore, we recommend the apology session only be implemented with a system that has overcome its chronic tendency to drop out of treatment, or one that is monitored closely.

Family Systems Factors

Family structure, style, and communication patterns all need to be addressed therapeutically and cannot be done so in brief therapy. For example, the family may display a rigidly enmeshed pattern of dysfunction, involving strict adherence to a patriarchal set of rules, and an intolerance of outside relationships. Hence, therapeutic interventions should include encouragement for the family to attempt alternative behaviors. These interventions can assume the form of homework assignments; enactments; insight-oriented questions; or any other intervention the clinician uses to effect change. An incestuous family's patterns of behaviors are very resistant to change and Trepper and Sprenkle (1989) recommend intervention on one dimension at a time. Trepper and Sprenkle (1989) provide an excellent case example illustrating specific ways or techniques through which this structural change can be achieved.

Some clinicians believe the power issues inherent in structural dysfunction should be addressed more directly. For example, Grunebaum (1987) states that power is often used to enforce unfair social arrangements and cannot be ignored; a therapist must address unequal power relations within a family to avoid being unfair. However, it is her conviction (and the conviction of contextual therapy) that this is best accomplished by addressing imbalances of fairness and the ensuing lack of trust that follows. Power tactics are viewed as a statement of despair about the possibilities of trust and trustworthiness, reciprocity, and negotiation (Grunebaum, 1987).

Taylor (1986) states that perpetrators commonly tend to desire and abuse power in their family relationships. Consequently, they must learn to express and share power within the family system. Commonly, incestuous clients are seen by family members as authoritarian tyrants who may use oppressive, overt tactics or manipulation and subtle coercion to compensate for inner feelings of helplessness and inadequacy; other clients express power and control needs more indirectly (Taylor, 1986). Conte (1986) asserts that sexual abuse of children by fathers inherently involves abuse of parental power and alignment of parental power should be a treatment goal. In addition, imbalances of power, control, and influence between partners in the marital dyad should be addressed when they are present.

Larson and Maddock (1986) discuss how treatments may differ depending upon whether the incest appears to be affection-based, erotic-based, aggression-based, or rage-based. They believe that these four categories can serve as guidelines for developing treatment approaches that are highly "coupled" with both the functional meanings and the structural characteristics of various incestuous families. For example, a highly confrontive program that focuses on identifying and exchanging anger between family members may be very useful to an aggression-based incest family, while the same treatment approach to an affection-based family may generate confusion, shame, anxiety and resistance since it will likely fail to address this family's experience in a meaningful way (Larson & Maddock, 1986).

Faulty communication patterns in the incestuous family can be addressed through direct in-session intervention. Many perpetrators can be seen as "alexithymic," that is, unable to express their feelings in words or age-appropriate behaviors. They have rarely identified, much less understood, many of their emotions, and therefore they inconsistently and often inappropriately express their feelings

(Taylor, 1986). Hence, recognition and verbal expression of feelings toward family members is an appropriate goal for family therapy. This may go hand in hand with the learning of empathetic concern for others (Taylor, 1986), although in our experience, families find it much more difficult to develop genuine empathy.

Family of Origin Factors

Many incest perpetrators have never dealt with their own experience as incest victims. In order for lasting change to occur, adults who were molested as children who become molesters themselves must deal with the trauma of their own molestation and realize its relationship to their adult, sexually deviant behavior (Taylor, 1986). Until the client's underlying feelings of pain, fear, anger, excitement, and guilt stemming from his own childhood molestation are actively released through therapy, the incestuous client remains at high risk to repeat his active victimization through molestation, regardless of other behavioral changes (Taylor, 1986).

Self-Help Groups

We advocate judicious use of self-help groups for both perpetrators and survivors. Such groups are beneficial insofar as they help the family extend external homeostatic mechanisms. Specific assistance may be received from support groups such as Parents Anonymous, Perpetrators Anonymous, Incestual Fathers Anonymous, or similar organizations, most of which are organized around Twelve-Step principles (Pardeck, 1989; Trepper & Barrett, 1986b). However, many of these groups do not appear as "ego sound" as a typical AA group and may encourage premature disclosure which they are ill-equipped to manage. We have occasionally needed to perform crisis intervention following attendance at self-help groups for incest, something we have never had to do for AA, NA, GA, or any other Twelve-Step related group. However, self-help groups are useful for crisis-prone victims or perpetrators as long as they remain basically supportive.

If alcohol is involved, a safer referral might be to AA first. At AA or its related family adjuncts, the client family can receive social support and also view a wider variety of healthier behaviors than they might in other settings. The ubiquitousness of AA also adds to its clinical utility. Finally, AA attendance seems to have a very powerful effect of reducing a variety of family resistances.

Individual Factors

The parents should be expected to progress in the areas of individual dysfunction that were encountered during the assessment phase. For example, if the therapist discovers in treatment that the mother has resentment toward the victim, these feelings need to be addressed in therapy (Taylor, 1986). Similarly, if the therapist finds that the father continues to blame the victim for the sexual abuse, treatment might then be concentrated on helping him accept responsibility for the sexual abuse and enhancing guilt feelings about what he has done. Alleviation of alcohol abuse is often a goal for the perpetrator and can be addressed either through self-help or through more formal treatment. Participation in drug treatment programs, in addition to family therapy, may be appropriate (Cornille, 1989). The promotion of healthy sexual desire, knowledge, and functioning is crucial in the treatment process and prevention of future molestation (Taylor, 1986). The sexual problems of the incest perpetrator are often underexplored and thereby undertreated by many professionals (Taylor, 1986). Along those lines, Conte (1986) states that we must be aware that sexual abuse of children is a complex problem involving, at least in part, sexual arousal and sexual fantasies involving children. Giaretto (1989) advocates a humanistic approach which focuses on elimination of feelings of self-hatred and a promotion of feelings of self-worth, thereby reducing likelihood of future treatment resistance.

Socio-Environmental Factors

The perpetrator must recognize the causes for his sense of isolation and the impact of this on behavior patterns. He must then move from isolation into adult social interaction. Although awareness is the first step in reducing the isolation of the perpetrator and his family, effective treatment must also include teaching, practicing, and reinforcement of new social skills (Taylor, 1986). Group treatment provides built-in opportunities for social experience and learning; however, group treatment cannot replace interaction with the wider social environment (Taylor, 1989). Goals might include expansion of the client's social network involving at least one active friendship outside the extended family, or expansion of both the couple and family social network, including at least two couple and family activities outside the home per month (Taylor, 1986).

Although it may not be part of the treatment plan for a particular family, clinicians should strive to influence community and societal practices that contribute to the perpetuation of incest. Among other things, primary prevention of incest depends on changes in attitudes toward sexuality and gender roles.

Precipitating Events

The nature of the precipitating event for the particular family determines upon whether it is an appropriate target for intervention. For example, consumption of alcohol is certainly an appropriate intervention target, whereas chronic physical illness of the mother is not. The latter case would be best managed by helping the family develop a means for coping with the effects of the mother's illness.

Coping Mechanisms

The positive social network the family develops may serve as a coping mechanism in and of itself (Trepper & Barrett, 1986b). Pardeck (1989) emphasizes the need to teach parents coping skills such as child, time, and home management techniques. The precise coping mechanisms that are taught will depend upon the stressors a particular family faces, as well as strengths of the family. Along these lines, the general teaching of problem-solving skills is often advocated (Taylor, 1986) and is usually very helpful with the resistant family.

CONCLUSION

The impact of incest on the abused child can be devastating (Giaretto, 1989). It is important that those responsible for dealing with incestuous families not let their anger at the offending parent blind them to methods for preventing future incest. Through coordinated intervention on a variety of different levels, it may be possible to restore even a resistant family to reasonably healthy functioning. Family therapy is a crucial part of this intervention, and it is hoped that this chapter provides some guidance to the family and crisis therapist.

Chapter Ten

Delinquency
and the Resistant Family

A common pattern observed in the treatment of the resistant family is for one or more children to be adjudicated by the legal system as delinquent. Court involvement often serves to mandate the otherwise treatment resistant family into ongoing therapy (Johnson, 1974), regardless of their preferences. Few situations are as frustrating to the family therapist as attempting to help the treatment resistant system when the sole client impetus for seeking professional help is to satisfy a court requirement. Furthermore, many of the techniques that we have advocated for treating the resistant family system are ineffectual in such situations. This chapter briefly reviews theory and intervention techniques useful for treating crisis-prone and resistant systems when the presenting problem is legal involvement of minors.

THE EFFICACY OF FAMILY THERAPY
WITH DELINQUENTS

Therapy with delinquent families constitutes some of the most challenging work the family therapist will confront. This is even more true when the delinquent is from a family system that is frequently in crisis and thwarts the therapist's best intentions. Throughout this volume we have advocated that such families cannot be forced to change. Instead, they should be given informed options regarding their behaviors and provided with the opportunity to try more functional coping strategies. However, as in cases of incest or child abuse, this philosophy is inappropriate when the family's presenting or compounding problem is delinquency. This is because the consequences of failure to change are severe and often permanent. The family-oriented crisis therapist will have to assume a more traditional therapeutic stance with delinquent families, a stance that may seem anti-intuitive to practitioners who are accustomed to working with families using brief models of therapy.

However, the treatment of delinquency is one of the few areas where family therapists can unequivocally regard their techniques as the treatment of choice. The issue of family treatment of delinquency has spawned a complex and voluminous literature. In terms of outcome research, Tolan, Cromwell, and Brasswell (1986) raised three questions: (1) Is there evidence that family therapy is effective with delinquents? (2) Is family therapy *more* effective than other approaches? and (3) What factors influence effectiveness? Each of these questions is important and will be discussed briefly.

These authors reviewed 34 chapters, books, and articles in an effort to address the evidence regarding efficacy of family therapy with delinquents. They concluded that extant studies provide general support for linking poor family functioning to the development of delinquency, and that family therapy intervention relates to improved family functioning with reduced delinquency. However, methodological concerns and the lack of comparative studies contrasting family therapy with other therapeutic modalities makes the conclusion regarding these linkages equivocal.

In order to address the second question, Tolan, Cromwell, and Brasswell (1986) identified and reviewed eight investigations that specifically compared family therapy with other types of intervention. These studies consistently reported family therapy to be more effective than other interventions in reducing delinquency. For example, two studies compared family therapy with individual therapy and both demonstrated family therapy to be more effective (Parsons & Alexander, 1973; Sutton, 1978). Similarly, Maskin (1976) demonstrated a community-oriented family treatment program in significantly less recidivism than a work-oriented program, and Stuart, Jayartone, and Tripodi (1976) found family therapy to be more effective than individually-oriented problem-solving training. Finally, Johnson (1977) compared structural/strategic family therapy with traditional probation services and found no significant difference in recidivism rates between the groups during the first year after treatment. However, during the second year, the recidivism rate for the probation group increased more than for the family therapy group.

Tolan, Cromwell, and Brasswell (1986) explored the factors influencing the effect of family therapy upon delinquents through reviewing investigations that examined the effects of different therapeutic modalities, therapist variables (technical skills vs. relationship skills), and characteristics of delinquents on successful versus unsuccessful family therapy outcome. Inconsistent results were found. However, these authors conclude that optimal treatment for delinquents consists of a combination of behavioral and structural/ strategic family therapy techniques within an intrafamilial communication focus, especially for first-time and status offenders.

Similarly, Ulrici (1983) reviewed the literature on effects of behavioral and family interventions on juvenile recidivism, and concluded that the *combination* of behavioral interventions with a family systems approach likely held the most promise for treatment of delinquency. However, this author raised the consideration that combined behavioral and systems theory interventions may not be more effective or cost efficient than working with the family system alone. Specifically, Ulrici offered four conclusions: (1) behavioral intervention applied without consideration of family dynamics can be effective in changing target behaviors but these treatment gains do not deter recidivism; (2) family interventions have been generally successful in lowering recidivism rates when compared to no-treatment and alternative treatment controls; (3) approaches combining behavioral techniques with family involvement were successful only when overall aspects of the family system were addressed; and (4) family therapies concerned with changing family dynamics but not utilizing behavioral techniques were as effective as those interventions combining behavioral and family systems approaches.

Overall, these studies support family therapy as the treatment of choice for problems of delinquency. Behavioral interventions may be useful adjuncts to family therapy, although data is less clear regarding this issue.

FAMILY FACTORS AND DELINQUENCY

The review of Tolan, Cromwell, and Brasswell (1986) provides an excellent point of departure for treatment of resistant delinquent families. These authors specify three common family systemic qualities that have been emphasized in the research regarding delinquency: (1) ineffective, contradictory, or inefficient parental skills or authority; (2) disjointed/unclear family communication (particularly around conflict resolution); and (3) the functional utility of the delinquent's behavior within the family. Each characteristic is important and will be discussed below.

Parenting Problems

Experience working with delinquent families suggests that families whose primary problems relate to ineffective, contradictory or inefficient parental authority are often excellent treatment candidates for short term intervention. Much of the success of family therapy in this area might relate to the fact that many families present primarily with this problem. In general, these families would not meet our definition of a resistant family. Instead, they may simply lack appropriate parenting skills and knowledge. Although they may gain access to the mental health system through encountering a crisis, they usually respond quite well to intervention. Often, they only need to receive brief consultation before they can solve their own problems. The Family Study below illustrates such a family.

Family Study 10.1. The Westport Family

Julia and Tom Westport were an African-American family living in the suburbs with their children Tania, 14, and J'wan, 10. Both parents worked arduous hours and the children were often left unsupervised. Neither parent had had an optimal—or for that matter, satisfactory—childhood. Both had come from homes where parental authority had been absolute, punative, and exceedingly capricious. In response to these experiences, Julia and Tom maintained an extremely lax attitude regarding household rules and restrictions.

When Tania was arrested for shoplifting, the parents blamed themselves for being too punitive and harsh. They relaxed the family's rules even more. Without any behavioral consequences being present in the home, Tania soon became involved in drugs. She was arrested for participating in a burglary with her boyfriend, which naturally prompted a severe family crisis.

Terms of Tania's probation mandated that the family receive ongoing therapy. The therapist was able to teach Tom and Julia about the need to parent in a consistent and limit-setting way. Although Tania greatly resented the abundance of new rules that came with therapy, she was able to "shape up" and had no more legal problems. On the most recent follow-up she was a sophomore in college and reported doing well. J'wan was also doing well, and had just been admitted to his high school honor society.

Communications Problems

In treating the resistant system, the latter two aspects of delinquent families discussed by Tolan, Cromwell, and Brasswell (1986), communications problems and homeostatic functionality of delinquency, assume the greatest importance. Presently much of the research into the dynamics of delinquent families continues to focus on communication variables and attributions. For example, Lipsitt, Lelos, and Gibbs (1985) characterized communication patterns in delinquent families as secretive, distorting, and hostile. They concluded the lack of a stable nurturant family setting combined with faulty communication patterns would appear to be "excellent" predictors of juvenile long-term involvement in delinquent behavior.

In another study on positive and negative family communication processes, Lessin and Jacob (1984) found that constructive communications in a conflict situation within normal families occurred through "multichannels" and contained both a negative verbal and a positive nonverbal component. They hypothesized that the positive nonverbal communication may serve to either soften the negative verbal message or to communicate approval and acceptance of the receiver while simultaneously communicating verbal disapproval with the receiver's behavior. Similarly, Barton et al. (1985) reviewed the research on behavioral correlates of dysfunctional communicational interaction in delinquent families, and their association between problematic cognitions. They found that delinquent families do not expect each other to comply with requests or demands, nor do they expect to be able to exert influence on each other unless they use "nonconventional" forms of communication.

Family Study 10.2 illustrates rather graphically the communications deficits delinquent families, especially resistant delinquent families, have. Note the way that the family communicates, or more accurately, fails to communicate, unless something obscene is said.

Family Study 10.2. The Staymakers

John Staymaker, 49, his girlfriend Pat, 42, and John's son Rex, 13, showed up unannounced at a local mental health clinic. The previous evening, Rex had been arrested for stealing a car. He was released on parental bond and returned home only to get into a fight with Pat. John announced to the crisis worker that he is "dumping this goddamn kid off with his mother" in another state. Upon hearing this, Rex rampaged through the family's apartment and destroyed as much furniture as he could until his father physically restrained him. The family has a history of periodic mental health involvement, usually focusing on the substance abuse of other siblings who are not present in the interview. (The transcript begins about 20 minutes into the crisis session).

Therapist: What do you think of what your father has said?

Rex: (Obviously distracted) Huh? Nothing. He's full of shit. As usual. He's fucked. I hope he dies.

Therapist: How's that?

Rex: He wants to tell me about how high and mighty he is and he won't even send my mother the support check. Fuck. Fuckin' right I'm mad. And I'm gonna keep fuckin' up until he pays my mother.

Therapist: Have you thought about telling him this? How you feel? Maybe what made you mad?

Rex: Hmm. (To father). Yeah. You're full of shit.

John: Shut up, you little bastard! Goddamn! You think you can . . .

Therapist: No, I mean, about the other part. About you being angry. (At this point Rex discusses his behavior. The father and Pat both ignore him and distractedly gaze out of the window).

Rex: (At the end of a long narrative, appropriate in tone and without profanity, which was also completely ignored) . . . . So you all can fuck yourselves. That's what I say . . . I mean it.

John: You see! He wants to know why I don't listen to him. And it's because all he does is curse. Look at him. Looks like he's sleeping. I'd like to beat the holy shit out of him. (Rex perks up immediately.)

Therapist: You know, it seems the only way anyone in this family gets anyone else's attention is to curse.

John: I don't know about that.

Frequently, families like these require lengthy treatment and are not amenable to brief, problem-oriented solutions. Moreover, delinquent families that communicate poorly are highly likely to have many perceptual crises. They often have a clinical history long before there is any active delinquency. On the other hand, families that lack parenting skills usually come in contact with mental health professionals only under court order.

Delinquency and Family Homeostasis

Another problem often encountered in resistant families is when delinquency seems to fulfil an important homeostatic function for the family system. Within the context of family homeostasis and delinquency, Johnson (1978) has proposed a specific and developed conceptualization of delinquency as a function of the family system. Applying concepts from strategic, structural, and contextual theories of family systems, Johnson maintains that delinquency serves as a family homeostatic device that signals a failing family system. This process brings aid to the family from extended family, social agencies, or the community, in an attempt to help the family cope with or reform the delinquent. He posits that the delinquent also organizes a dysfunctional family system by becoming the scapegoat for the family. Consequently, the delinquent behavior provides a problem that can ally disengaged parents, induce parents to reclaim previously abdicated authority, and mobilize family members to form a cohesive unit organized around their efforts to rehabilitate and/or blame the delinquent.

The Family Study below highlights the way that family members sometimes employ delinquency to maintain homeostasis.

Family Study 10.3. The Blakes

Captain John Blake, 46, was a reservist called to active duty as part of Operation Desert Shield. His marriage to Marion, 43, was shaky at best. The couple quarreled frequently and had sexual difficulties. Moreover, Marion began to wonder about her preferred gender orientation for this phase of her life. While John was in Saudi Arabia, she became sexually involved with a same gender friend who recently had come "out."

As the affair became known among the couple's children, each reacted intensely. John Jr., 14, got into "legal trouble," a series of home robberies occurring when he should have been in school. The family tension rose to the point that Marion decided that she had to "break off" with her lover "until things clear up at home."

Once he returned home Captain Blake suggested marital therapy. Marion rejected this idea because she had no interest in continuing the relationship. When the couple was just about ready to separate, their next child, Steven, 12, was arrested for breaking windows of unoccupied buildings. Concern over the two boys kept the couple together, at least temporarily.

In the experience of many clinicians, treatment resistance in delinquent families is usually related to the homeostatic function delinquency serves for the family system. Families who employ delinquency as a device to preserve intimacy, family unity, or autonomy are particularly likely to sabotage any therapeutic regimen imposed by an outside agent. Families may then abruptly report their problems as "solved" or "cured" and summarily terminate treatment. If outside stressors escalate, then family cohesion may decrease and the family may again be at risk for future delinquency to restabilize the family system.

When dysfunctional homeostatic mechanisms are superimposed on communications deficits, the clinical picture of the classic resistant family emerges: a family that is both crisis-prone (from poor communications) and treatment resistant (due to the functional aspects of the delinquency on the family system). Because of the unique factors operating to make the system treatment resistant and crisis-prone, brief therapy is practically useless when the family demonstrates both communications problems and delinquency-related homeostasis.

TREATING THE RESISTANT DELINQUENT FAMILY

Our strategy for working with the delinquent family is to treat them symptomatically. We evaluate and assess parenting skills, communications problems, homeostatic mechanisms, and other relevant family areas. We then adjust our interventions according to whatever problems we find. Treatment is problem focused rather than theoretically driven. Interventions may range from behavioral and structural, to interpretive and psychodynamic, depending upon what seems appropriate to the problem at hand.

As stated above, poor parental skills are rarely the sole problem of a family system that is treatment resistant and crisis-prone. However, many delinquent families show profound deficits in parenting ability. Often, these aspects are the easiest to change and sometimes merely proper information and education may dispel significant ignorance. There are several excellent texts regarding the teaching of parenting skills. Many behavior-oriented family therapy approaches are useful in treating skills deficits. Link therapists, discussed in Chapter Eight, also can be effective regarding acquisition of specific parental behaviors.

Communication Problems of Delinquent Families

Perceptual crises in the delinquent family system are often kindled by communications related to conflict or conflict resolution. Families with poor communication patterns are typically crisis-prone, particularly when delinquency is the presenting problem. Because of this factor, treatment of the delinquent family should always include an assessment of the family's ability to communicate. In those cases with severe communications deficits, a longer-term and therapeutic stance is often necessary, as opposed to a consultational mode.

Family communications problems are frequently more clinically dramatic than homeostatic dysfunctioning. Thus, they are usually evident during the first family interview, even when the family presents during a crisis. Such families will have extraordinary difficulties staying within the guidelines of crisis therapy rules discussed in Chapter Five. For example, the entire family may talk at once to the therapist and may not be able to talk to each other at all.

One cognitive behavioral technique we have found useful with delinquent families is that of reframing the delinquent family's causal attributions. Inherent in this intervention is the conceptualization that the actual content of verbalizations in delinquent families is not as important as family member assumptions that communications contain content designed to exploit, hurt, or antagonize other family members. The emphasis here is on attributional processes in disturbed relationships and on cognitive-based therapeutic maneuvers emphasizing nonblaming and positive interpretation of family communications, issues, and symptoms. The goal of the therapy lies in teaching the family to listen to what is being said and, whenever possible, attribute a positive meaning to the verbal content.

Examples of these types of interventions are presented by Barton et al., (1985), and Alexander, Waldron, Barton, and Mas, (1989). These authors advocate concentrating on a family's attributional framework and emphasizing the positive aspects of family life and communications during early therapeutic interactions. Positive interpretation or reframing is used to modify family members' perceptions or attributions regarding other family members and problems, thus indirectly enhancing positive communications. Barton et al. acknowledge there is very little empirical support for these clinical techniques and assertions. However, those author's experiences and our own clinical experience suggest they are helpful, especially in the early stages of therapy with the resistant family.

A further advantage of enhancing positive attributions regarding communication is that they may reduce family resistance. For example, Alexander, Waldron, Barton, & Mas (1989) note that initial focus on nonblaming, relational aspects of the delinquent's behavior and motivations may enable the therapist to decrease expressions of resistance typically encountered in these families. In contrast, initial focus on problems may elicit higher rates of negative attributions and behaviors which are not easily modified.

Other authors have recommended behavioral solutions to increasing the quality and quantity of family communications. For example, contingency contracting regarding communications issues is popular with some therapists. This technique is particularly useful with the multiproblematic family. Contingency contracts have two functions: (1) to schedule exchange of major reinforcements known to reduce frequency and intensity of arguments over how and when reinforcements are to be exchanged; and (2) requires parents to cooperate since they must agree on behavioral expectations and consequences. In this method, family problems are defined, members express how they feel about each problem, and family coping methods and limitations are assessed. At this point, new coping methods are then introduced and practiced. Use of more effective coping methods is thought to decrease family tension and disorganization, factors believed to contribute to delinquency.

Delinquent families may be at greater risk to misperceive nonverbal communications (McCown, Johnson, & Austin, 1986). Certain families have extensive deficits necessitating basic remedial interventions to teach them how to differentiate facial or bodily expressions. In these situations, role playing and rote rehearsal of emotional discrimination can be useful. For example, delinquent families that consistently misunderstand each other's nonverbal communications may require direct exposure to and practice in the skills needed to differentiate emotional and facial expressions of disgust, anger, or surprise.

Sometimes, the therapist finds that he or she is the sole mechanism through which the resistant and delinquent family can plan joint behavior or communicate sensitive feelings. When this is the case, the therapist may first intervene with time-limited treatment so the family will work harder to build self-reliance. In more severe cases, therapy may never overcome the need for each session to provide crisis intervention and ego lending to family members. This is particularly likely when the family has a long history of dysfunction, is of lower intelligence or undereducated, or has multiple members with demonstrated antisocial behaviors.

Delinquent families will frequently terminate treatment upon enhancement of communication effectiveness because they may view their problem as solved and see no more need for therapy. This is especially likely if treatment has been slow or gains have been painfully secured through great effort. As is the case with most crisis-prone and treatment resistant families, it is generally not useful to force such families into continued treatment. Effort should be expended to sensitize the family to the possibility they may wish to return to treatment "after a vacation," or they may require a "booster" session in the future. Naturally, the door should always remain open to seeing these families quickly once they decide to return for additional therapy.

Enhancing Family Homeostasis

Hypothesized homeostatic dysfunctions within the family system can be demonstrated either through observation or formal systemic assessment using one of several diagnostic instruments. For example, Maynard and Hultquist (1988) report successful utilization of the Circumplex Model of Ohlson and his associates. Families that are enmeshed or disengaged are prime candidates for the therapist's hypothesis that delinquent behavior holds a functional aspect for the family system. However, the veracity of this hypothesis cannot be established until the clinician has observed an example of this behavioral syndrome. This constitutes another reason why the therapy of delinquents is often of long-term duration. It is not until the behavior is observed during family treatment that the therapist and the family can explore it further.

Behavior that is dysfunctional for the family system may have positive aspects for other systems. This is stressed in the theory and treatment methodology of practitioners of family-ecological systems approaches advocated by Henggeler et al. (1986). They propose that in contrast with most family therapies, the family-ecological systems approach best addresses the multidimensional nature of behavior problems. They note that there are many instances in which transactions within the child's extrafamilial systems, (i.e., peer group, school, or individual factors, or poor social skills or problem-solving strategies), are more critical determinants of problem behavior than family relations. Therefore, treatment is focused upon the identified dysfunction in a system or between two or more systems, with emphasis on changing transactions between and among pertinent systems. The specific treatments offered to the families range from structural to behavioral.

Recent research efforts appear to be directed largely towards developing and implementing family therapy interventions involving systems other than the family (Atkinson & McKenzie, 1987; Henggeler et al., 1986; Burford & Casson, 1989; Gordon, Arbuthnot, Gustafson, & McGreen, 1988; Kagan, Reid, Roberts, & Silverman-Pollow, 1987; Lipsitt, Lelos, & Gibbs, 1985; Maynard & Hultquist, 1988). An implicit theoretical underpinning of these interventions is the notion the family's homeostatic mechanisms are permanently damaged and stability needs to be gained through interaction with other systems. Hence, many of these interventions require cooperation with the juvenile probation department, corrections personnel, children and youth social services, and the school system. Needless to say, this is often time-consuming for the therapist, and cooperation is often difficult to obtain.

If the therapist believes that the homeostatic function of delinquent behavior is perpetuating the cycle of delinquency, treatment should generally proceed with the goals advocated elsewhere in this volume for treating resistant systems. For example, the Hill/ McCubbin ABC-X model provides useful guidance for intervention focus. Knowledge for where to intervene is essential inasmuch as external stressors may need to be identified and limited, or other undefined variables may be operating. Often, the therapist must ego-lend to the family in order to assist in identification of the nature and extent of life stressors. Family perceptions of stressors and causal attributions may also require assessment and subsequent modification.

Functional coping should be modeled and consistently suggested to the family. Substance abuse as a coping mechanism may be especially problematic and command the majority of treatment efforts. Establishment of appropriate community supports by the resistant family should also be a treatment priority. If at all possible, the family should be encouraged to develop appropriate self-help and religious peer supports, although this is often more difficult with the delinquent family than with the other resistant systems.

As with most resistant families, a return to normalcy following a crisis period is often associated with a "honeymoon phase." The system believes it is permanently cured and consequently sees no reason for further treatment. This is often exacerbated by the fact that dysfunctional coping mechanisms work very quickly to return the family to baseline functioning following a crisis. If this happens, the delinquent family will terminate, only to return when there is another crisis.

Because of this some practitioners prefer to maintain a degree of family destabilization during the treatment so that the system does not terminate prematurely. Obviously, this should never be done during a crisis situation. Furthermore, attempts to destabilize the family system need to be pursued with extreme caution, since the system has already demonstrated the tenacity with which criminal or antisocial behavior maintains family equilibrium. We rarely recommend this technique when the IP presents with a history of increasingly dangerous delinquency. As with all resistant families, attempts to destabilize the system are also potentially dangerous due to the fact that the family may abruptly terminate treatment at any time. When working with delinquent families who have a history of treatment noncompliance it is often helpful to pretend as if each session is the last, thereby limiting the number of interventions that may prove problematic if the family decides to terminate without notice.

CONCLUSION

Practitioners who treat families are handicapped by the fact that such families may abruptly terminate treatment, even under court supervision. The practitioner must carefully balance the long-term needs of the family with the realization that treatment compliance cannot be assumed. Brief, empowering therapeutic approaches will probably prove ineffective. Initial successes may encourage over-confidence and subsequent abrupt termination. Dysfunctional coping styles may change slowly, if at all. Hence, brief therapy may be desirable, yet simultaneously impossible. Progress at changing structural problems within the system may occur sporadically, and in some cases may be impossible to obtain, at least with our current methods of family intervention.

Chapter Eleven

Families of
Brain-Compromised Individuals

It is unknown how many treatment resistant families contain members with organic brain impairment. However, the role of cognitive deficits in causing or contributing to resistance is an area of empirical inquiry that clearly needs additional attention. Clinical experience suggests that at least a subset of resistant systems function poorly because specific members lack the cognitive capacity to problem solve and/or remain in treatment. Many of these deficits are quite subtle, and perhaps undetectable in the absence of sophisticated neuropsychological and neuroimaging techniques. Others, such as those following major head injury, are quite obvious.

The purpose of this chapter is to discuss interventions that can assist the family of the brain-compromised patient in coping, adjustment, and reestablishing family equilibrium. As in cases of incest and delinquency, the techniques advocated for treating the resistant family are often inappropriate for this subgroup of families, due to the nature of the IP's status. Moreover, the therapist/consultant who works with families of individuals who have experienced cognitive impairment often have the opportunity to *prevent* a system from acquiring resistant characteristics. A focus on the unique difficulties faced by these families will serve to decrease the probability that brain-compromised individuals and their families will become crisis-prone and treatment resistant.

THE BRAIN-COMPROMISED:
A GROWING POPULATION

For various reasons, the past two decades have seen a dramatic increase in individuals who survive traumatic brain injury only to experience a moderate to severe degree of compromise in brain function. As medical science and sophisticated technology expands the capacity to preserve life, many thousands of young people who experience brain trauma are saved. Similarly, millions of elderly who might have succumbed to previously untreatable maladies find their lives extended, sometimes by decades. The growing number of elderly in the United States and in Europe, coupled with known incidence rates of dementia (cognitive decline), virtually guarantees that many more people will experience some degree of cognitive impairment within their life span. The effects of alcoholism and chronic substance abuse also contribute significantly to the increase in persons who must live with and adjust to brain compromise (McCown & Johnson, 1991). Finally, the cognitive deficits and ensuing consequences of neurotropic infections such as HIV disease are now beginning to be realized, with the individual effects of brain compromise yet to be fully established.

Many of these brain-compromised individuals or their families will seek some form of mental health service, rehabilitation, or contact with professional practitioners. Unfortunately, most mental health clinicians lack the training and specialized experience necessary to fully understand the complexities involved in treating these patients. Crisis intervention and therapy with families of brain-compromised individuals is an intricate area encompassing neurology, neuropsychology, personality theory, psychiatry, social services, and family systems theory. No single discipline or profession contains sufficient expertise in all of these areas. However, we believe that an understanding of the systemic factors involved in this type of family adaptation is essential for clinicians who wish to effectively assist these individuals.

For purposes of illustration and discussion, brain-compromised individuals can be roughly divided into two major groups. This is not meant to imply that brain-compromised individuals are homogeneous with respect to the course of their difficulty inasmuch as many factors account for degree of cognitive impairment and ensuing adjustment. Rather, the purpose is to facilitate understanding of the diversity of brain-compromise while demonstrating common problems confronted within the individual and the family unit.

The first group consists of individuals with closed head injury, usually from traumatic brain insult, and the second group is composed of individuals who suffer from dementia with varying etiologies, but primarily from degenerative disorders or Alzheimer's disease. Through the use of case illustrations, each group will be discussed in terms of age, nature of onset of brain dysfunction, individual and family dynamics, and problems typically encountered in these families. A theoretical developmental framework for conceptualizing individual and familial adjustment to brain-compromised individuals will be presented, and family therapy strategies in the context of this developmental progression will be presented.

TRAUMATIC BRAIN INJURY

Individuals with traumatic brain injury are likely between the ages of 15 to 25, and alcohol or drug abuse has been implicated in approximately half of these cases. A typical case might present as follows.

Family Study 11.1. The O'Donnells

A 23-year-old divorced secretary (oldest of two children) who had moved back in with her family of origin was struck by a car and dragged over 100 feet as she exited a party and attempted to cross a major highway. She required resuscitation on the site, had multiple abrasions and internal injuries, and a compressed skull fracture in the left frontal area. She was transported to the nearest emergency room for treatment, and a CT Scan indicated the presence of diffuse contusions. Eventually, she required neurosurgery to relieve her brain of pressure related to her injury.

Her parents and younger sister (16 years old) were awakened in the middle of the night by a phone call from the police officer who responded to the scene of the accident and advised them to come immediately to the hospital. Worried, they quickly dressed, and her father grumbled that he could not miss an important meeting in the morning. The parents were met at the hospital by the security guard who directed them to the surgical intensive care unit (SICU) where the patient had been transferred from the emergency room. When the parents and younger sister were allowed into the SICU, they saw their daughter, deeply comatose, grotesquely disfigured, and on a respirator. She had multiple facial and bodily lacerations, and her entire head was swollen. She remained comatose for two weeks, and had a period of confusion (known as post-traumatic amnesia) for close to six weeks as she was coming out of her coma.

Once the patient was stabilized medically, she was transferred to a residential rehabilitation facility for eight months. Ambulatory, she had cognitive deficits including lack of short-term memory and a frontal lobe syndrome when she was discharged to the care of her parents. Briefly, features of frontal lobe brain-compromise include cognitive concreteness, difficulties initiating activities, problems in sequencing steps to reach a certain goal, generalized slowing of responses and thought processes, and behavioral passivity. Prognostically, she was able to care for basic needs, but was unlikely to be able to work in the future.

In this case, the issues confronting the family are typically overwhelming, unpredictable, and frightening. When the onset of cerebral injury is abrupt, a conceptual framework for the developmental progression of the family may be visualized as illustrated in Figure 11.1.

Note that this model begins with an abrupt onset, and outlines the progression of familial reactions as the individual proceeds through recovery from traumatic brain injury. Using the terminology of this volume, the family experiences a profound and shattering instrumental crisis. As in all extreme instrumental crises, immediate concerns involve the pragmatic, day-to-day disruption of normal routines as the family scrambles to accommodate this tragedy into their lives. Emotionally, shock and disbelief are likely to prevail. Those family members who are employed must juggle work responsibilities with bedside vigils, consultation with hospital staff, and suddenly planning for someone else's future. Immediate practical con-

FIGURE 11.1. Stages of Family Response to Traumatic Brain Injury

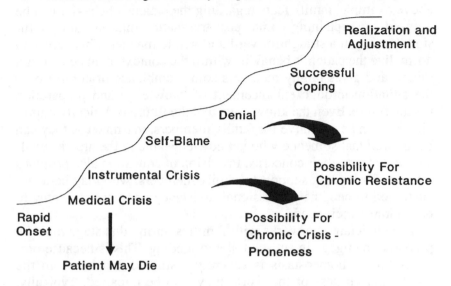

cerns are superimposed upon shock and grief, as well as a plethora of feelings that may include guilt reactions, self-blame, and sadness. Concern about the brain-injured individual may range from fears of imminent death to anger concerning pre-accident behavior. Hence, the family is in crisis as members attempt to assimilate new and frightening information amidst emotional upheaval.

Following the model established by our research group, we advocate that family interventions at this point be primarily focused upon defusing the tremendous tension precipitated by this type of crisis. With the possible exception of a sudden death, there is no crisis where it is more appropriate than traumatic brain injury to allow the family the chance to simply ventilate their concerns. As long as the patient remains medically unstable, it cannot be reasonably expected that the family will progress beyond this stage. In other words, it is usually inappropriate to proceed beyond the *D* in our "ADEPT" model. Evaluation, problem solving and translation will have to wait until the patient and the family have achieved some degree of stability.

A helpful strategy to defuse tension is to provide information and education concerning the typical course of acute brain injury. In the above example, family fears regarding the patient's behavior can be defused by explaining coma, post-traumatic amnesia, and confusional states in a straightforward and gentle manner. This serves to normalize the patient's behavior within the context of an acute brain injury, and gives family members some semblance of control over the situation through enhancement of knowledge and preparation for the future. Even the knowledge that the future is typically unpredictable can be palliative for family members, inasmuch as they can be assured that someone who is knowledgeable in the area is available to listen to their concerns. Provision of education also provides a forum for lending support to family members, who may be unaccustomed to needing professional assistance and uncertain how to best address their needs.

The clinician who works with families during this stage must be prepared to engage in substantial ego-lending. This is because previous family homeostasis is severely disrupted and belief in the equity and fairness of the world may also be impaired. Typically, coping mechanisms are overwhelmed, and even formerly effective strategies are usually not viable in such a novel and emotional disruptive situation. Consequently, the family may experience difficulty making some very basic decisions regarding the patient without extensive therapeutic support.

Often, families who experience acute traumatic brain injury will engage in unrealistic denial as they progress through the initial stage of shock and disbelief. As is sometimes the case with terminally ill individuals, these families may bargain with God or other Higher Power. Or, certain members may spend time speculating on "what ifs," such as what would the passage of one more minute prior to the accident have meant to the patient? They may also lapse into deep depression.

One way families will often attempt to return the overwhelmed family system to homeostasis is by exacerbating internally dysfunctional homeostatic mechanisms. Psychodynamically oriented clinicians have observed this for years and have labelled the phenomena as "acting out." The premise is that under conditions of family stress another family member displays the neurotic conflicts the family is fearful of verbalizing.

In our view, this phenomena is more usefully conceptualized through viewing the family members as unconsciously attempting to ventilate pressure accumulating on the family system. In this manner, somewhat crudely, the chance the family will survive is maximized. The Family Study below illustrates this common occurrence.

Family Study 11.2. The Smith Family

Regina Smith was the 12-year-old sister of John, 17, who had recently been involved in a serious accident and suffered traumatic brain injury.

During the long vigil that marked the gradual recovery of John, Regina became increasingly hostile and sullen. Five months after the accident she began drinking heavily and associating with an older, drug-oriented crowd.

Regina's parents expressed their concern regarding this change in behavior to their son's physician. The physician recommended that Regina be treated for alcohol abuse at a private inpatient facility. Because the parents could not afford this option, they sought additional consultation. A hospital social worker of analytic persuasion interviewed Regina and suggested that she receive psychodynamic psychotherapy to help her "relieve unexpressed feelings and gain emotional insight" regarding her brother's accident. This was tried for six weeks and terminated when Regina showed up intoxicated to one of the sessions.

A referral was then made to a family-oriented colleague who determined that Regina's problem was that the family system had abdicated its responsibility to her regarding the setting of necessary limits. Strategic interventions and paradoxes were invoked and Regina's parents became appropriately more mindful of her whereabouts. However, Regina continued to be sullen, angry, and increasingly impulsive. She also became bulimic on occasion.

Consultation was requested with a third social worker specializing in family adaptation following head injury. The social worker surmised that the family's disruption following

John's injury and the subsequent attention afforded exclusively to John had jeopardized Regina's feelings that her family cared for her. The social worker suggested that the family simply take some time off from John's recovery and resume some of their previous family activities.

The family reluctantly followed this advice, feeling quite a bit of guilt. They began to go shopping for necessities together for the first time since John's accident. They next began eating at home, instead of grabbing every meal at the hospital cafeteria. They finally resumed church attendance and participation in the junior high school swim team.

Within a few weeks Regina became more cooperative and less impulsive. She later stated that "I feel like I finally have my family back together."

As time progresses, coping strategies become manifest as family members strive for personal normalcy and order in their lives. For example, daily bedside vigils may give way to return to work and visiting the hospital nightly. Some family members may continue to attempt to cope through denial or conscious attempts to avoid thinking about the situation. Others may overcompensate and immerse themselves in the patient, sometimes to the exclusion of employment or other familial responsibilities. Still others may cope through avoidance of the patient or situation, and attempt to distance themselves from core familial concerns.

All of these coping strategies have implications for the family system and homeostasis in the sense they are superimposed upon pre-morbid factors both within the brain-compromised individual and the family functioning as a unit. The fact that individuals have unique coping styles and patterns of returning to personal normalcy often provides fertile ground for familial conflict. For example, in the above-outlined case, Regina may next attempt to cope through avoidance and over-involvement in activities related to school and friends. Her mother, on the other hand, may overcompensate through immersion in the patient's condition and progress to the relative neglect of other family members. Meanwhile, her father may react through emotional detachment and avoidance of the patient or situation. This interaction of individual coping styles, coupled with stressors inherent in the situation, may propel the family towards dysfunction, misunderstanding, and a cycle of frequent crises and treatment resistance.

The phase of realization and adjustment is typically when major assimilation and working through of the event can occur. Family members, despite various coping styles, must come to growing realization that the brain-compromised individual is not the same as before. That is, brain-compromise has typically resulted in both subtle and overt behavioral, emotional, and personality changes.

Along these lines, Lezak (1986) identified four clusters of difficulties commonly found in the brain-compromised individual. First, the individual may have impaired social perception and social awareness. A person with a significant personality change as a result of brain damage can display marked egocentricity coupled with diminished self-awareness. This puts the family unit under duress and strain inasmuch as the patient's behavior may become inappropriately demanding, self-centered, unreasonable, illogical, or unrealistic. For example, one family of a brain-compromised individual with subsequent reading impairment refused to eat out at restaurants because the individual insisted that the entire menu be read to him prior to ordering. This lack of self-awareness can also result in deceased capacity to be socially sensitive and considerate of the needs of others. Hence, the caretaker or family is confronted with a constant burden of demands, and frequently the social circle of such families decreases. Furthermore, resentment and anger can accumulate as each member (including the IP) feels misunderstood and "put upon."

A second difficulty identified by Lezak concerns impaired control which is usually manifest in impulsivity. This includes such behaviors as angry outbursts, overeating, sexual promiscuity, and excessive drinking. Conversely, impaired control can be manifest in difficulties in initiation or inhibition of spontaneous behavior. Unable to formulate goals and implement the necessary steps to achieving goals, these individuals often rely upon family members to provide structure and organize their behavior. They may also be concrete in thought and prone to literal interpretations of their environment, resulting in an excessive need for order and routine. Family members who disrupt such routine may suffer consequences of angry outbursts, or may instead find themselves locked into a fixed daily routine simply for the sake of the patient's rigidity. For example, one brain-compromised individual routinely insisted that her parents outline plans for the next day in explicit detail. This occurred every night, and if the parents refused to provide the information, or had not made plans for the next day, the individual would sulk or become very angry. On a rational level, the parents felt guilty for not honoring the request because they realized the individual was brain-injured and needed the information. On the other hand, they were angry at their forced role as organizers of the environment, and at being compelled to engage in such a nightly ritual.

A third group of difficulties surrounds the issue of dependence versus independence. An adult who sustains brain-compromise may have varying degrees of dependency, either of an emotional or physical nature. Reduced capacity for independent behavior often means the parents or caretaker have to take charge of components of the individual's life. This often unexpected responsibility may overwhelm or depress the caretaker, especially if they are older or retired.

Finally, Lezak identified specific emotional alterations that frequently occur in brain-compromised individuals and include anxiety, paranoia, and depression. The presence of cognitive deficits coupled with emotional changes can present a situation that is extremely demoralizing for family members. Cognitive difficulties in reasoning and judgment often impede the brain-compromised individual's ability to modulate emotional experience. At the same time, a family member may have difficulty reasoning with the upset member who is lacking in cognitive capability to "listen to reason." When an individual has managed to survive traumatic brain injury and requires a lengthy rehabilitation process, it is often particularly discouraging to family members that the brain-compromised individual sustains emotional changes concomitant to all other sequelae of brain injury. Families involved in the stage of realization and adjustment typically make frequent use of crisis mental health services. These families may also be treatment resistant for a variety of reasons that may be unknown to the clinician. Most often, a safe working hypothesis is that one or more family members is overinvolved with the patient's recovery. Other family members feel resentful and may try to avoid or even sabotage any regular mental health interventions aimed at enhancing the family's coping. The process of living through the recovery of a head trauma patient may therefore turn normally functioning families into resistant systems.

We feel that it is critical for the family therapist and other caregivers to encourage the family to develop autonomous problem-solving strategies regarding its changed member. The consultational role that we have seen as helpful in dealing with resistant families can empower the family while simultaneously decreasing dependency on the mental health professional. For example, during the coping stage we prefer to provide education and suggest options but not to make decisions for the family. This approach is advocated for several reasons. First of all, decisions are often required that have long-term effects and consequences for both the individual and family. The therapist must assist the family in formulating educated choices, but the ultimate responsibility and consequences for such decisions reside within the family. Secondly, each brain injury or insult presents a unique constellation of changes that are likely to evolve with the passage of time. Hence, the family must be equipped with a framework for viewing these changes and adjustment for a time span that usually includes several years, and feasibility of contact with a professional for such a prolonged time span is unlikely.

This role for the therapist may seem to be self-evident and a common practice. Often it is not. Families in this stage of recovery may literally beg the therapist to intervene inappropriately for them. They may act childishly or impulsively. They frequently display intense anger at the therapist who insists that the family maintain its autonomy. Often, it is tempting for the therapist to make decisions for the family rather than to cope with their constant inquiries, demands, and insecurities.

During this stage of recovery various family members often become preoccupied with "doing the right thing" for their damaged member. Simultaneously, many of the medical decisions that have been made regarding their member's care have been without familial input. As a result of this, the family may develop the classic learned helplessness that typifies other types of traumatized families. Minor stresses may prove intolerable. The family may begin to react inappropriately to daily events and seek crisis intervention for a variety of mundane perceptual crises. The therapist that does not empower the family to attempt to solve their own problems will soon see an overly dependent family system seeking therapeutic answers to insolvable dilemmas.

In earlier chapters, we have maintained that it is often helpful to tell the family that it is okay to make mistakes, and to avoid tendencies to be overly self-critical. This framework is consistent with the notion that the changed individual represents a novel challenge inasmuch as behavioral, emotional, and cognitive changes are dynamic and evolutionary in nature. We find this process of normalization extremely useful for families during this period of realization and adjustment. In the area of rehabilitation there are rarely any inviolate absolutes. Families usually respond well to an approach emphasizing the normalcy of an often trial-and-error approach with an individual whose cerebrally-induced idiosyncracies are not fully identified nor developed. Along these lines the therapist may need to develop and support the family's tolerance for ambiguity, and normalize the unpredictability of the situation.

The final phase of a family's development is that of acceptance and reintegration of the brain-compromised person into the family system. Family members no longer harbor unrealistic hopes for change or improvement, and have come to know the brain-compromised individual's idiosyncracies and eccentricities. At the same time, family members have accepted that the individual they knew prior to the accident effectively no longer exists, and that this "new" individual will need a new or different role in the family system. True reintegration of the individual can only occur once family members have identified and accepted emotional, personality, or behavioral changes. Former patterns of relating are gradually replaced with patterns dictated by the realities of the present and constraints of the future. New patterns of interaction perpetuate new memories and perspectives, and the brain-compromised individual is increasingly viewed for what he or she has become, as opposed to how he or she used to be. It is often during this period that family members may fully grieve their loss at the same time they attempt to accept the changed individual.

During this period we find linkage of family with community supports to be crucial. In many communities, a number of self-help organizations exist to assist the family in this transition. Referral can be made to these groups from the first day of the recovery process. However, families may reject such referrals as long as they foster unrealistic hopes regarding the patient's recovery. Later on, when the family is confronted with the daily problems of managing the changed family member, the system is usually much more open to accepting the help of nonprofessional community support.

If the patient's accident was drug or alcohol related, Alcoholics Anonymous (AA) or similar groups can prove invaluable. As we have stated throughout this volume, AA is often a useful modality for expanding the patient's social network, as well as discouraging the return to substance abuse that often accompanies physical, emotional, and cognitive recovery. AA or similar groups are also useful in helping the family establish some existential or spiritual meaning for the patient's trauma, which may facilitate acceptance. The family therapist who works with traumatic brain injury does well to maintain informal or formal liaisons with substance-related self-help groups in the community.

DEGENERATIVE DEMENTIA

Degenerative dementia results in brain-compromise in approximately 10 percent of Americans over the age of 65. A typical case may present as follows.

Family Study 11.3. The Maguires

The daughter and husband of a 73-year-old woman, Christine Maguire, have increasingly noticed her progressive memory loss, redundancies in speech, and momentary confusion. The family was referred to a neurologist, who conducted an examination and laboratory studies which were all negative. The family was then referred to a neuropsychologist, who conducted in-depth cognitive assessment. The patient, upon interview, insisted that nothing was wrong with her and demanded that the family mind their own business and allow her to continue handling her own finances. Privately, she revealed her notion that the family was plotting against her and wanted to see her committed in order to steal her money. The neuropsychologist determined the patient was suffering from Alzheimer's disease, an incurable degenerative disturbance which impairs cognition and often precipitates personality and emotional changes.

A developmental conceptualization of the family reaction to an individual with a dementing process can be graphically presented as in Figure 11.2. Note that this model includes an onset of brain-compromise that is gradual, progressive, and initially subtle. The individual is most cognitively intact at the beginning, until the gradual decline associated with dementia renders them progressively less able to reason, remember, or care for themselves.

Initially, the insidious onset of degenerative dementia promotes ambiguity and a familial search for explanations for memory loss or confusion. Complicating the situation is the fact that many individuals with early or mild dementia often rationalize or make excuses for their decreasing cognitive acumen. Capacity for self-awareness is typically affected, with resulting inability to self-critique and realize the presence of cognitive difficulties. This tendency to rationalize or lack self-awareness concerning cognitive deficits is complicated by the fact the individual often appears to be in control and does not superficially appear to experience difficulty. In both instances, family members are concerned but tend to minimize the cognitive decline, or attribute it to stressful events or the effects of normative aging. Many family members will deny outright that any significant changes are occurring, and insist that the affected individual is simply having a bad week. Hence, both affected individuals and family members are highly treatment resistant. Often, the individual may receive a neurological or neuropsychological evaluation indicating the objective presence of memory deficits (relative to standardized norms), suggestive of Alzheimer's disease. Frequently, professional feedback concerning this possibility, although often discounted by family members, contributes to the second phase of familial reaction, that of growing realization.

FIGURE 11.2. Five Stages of Family Coping Associated with Degenerative Brain Compromise

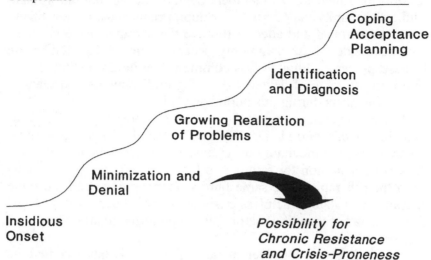

Coping
Acceptance
Planning

Identification
and Diagnosis

Growing Realization
of Problems

Minimization and
Denial

Insidious
Onset

*Possibility for
Chronic Resistance
and Crisis-Proneness*

    Growing realization that something is seriously wrong with the individual's cognitive functioning may be precipitated by behavior that is so completely out of character that it cannot be easily explained. For example, one family of a woman with early onset of Alzheimer's disease who had appeared to be managing reasonably well discovered she had not been paying her bills when her electricity was cut off. Another family was confronted with a similar situation when their elderly mother, who resided in a retirement home, was noted by the staff to neglect paying her rent. Frequently, this growing realization contributes to apprehension regarding the future of the demented individual, and each family member is confronted with considerations related to planning for another's future. Often at this point, if a neurological or neuropsychological evaluation has not occurred, the family will seek out such consultation, and a diagnosis of degenerative dementia will likely be made.

    The family is most likely to be crisis-prone at this period in the process. The family may seek out numerous experts to attempt to "fix" their impaired member, or generate a different or "correct" diagnosis. Each unusual or bizarre behavioral manifestation may spark a perceptual crisis among members that observe it. Family tension may increase, as members begin to accept the unfortunate truth. The family may argue over appropriate management of the impaired member and attempt to have the therapist arbitrate these disputes. Elder abuse commonly occurs during this period in the disease process. Although less common than in cases of traumatic brain injury, some of degree of "acting out" may also be seen by family members during this period as well.

A firm, empathetic, but realistic stance is most helpful for families during this period. Denial, a principal dysfunctional coping mechanism, will inevitably be associated with treatment resistance. It is not uncommon for families to break five or six appointments with their therapist. The same family members may call the same therapist in a state of helpless crisis only a few hours or days later! Patience, rather than limit-setting, is the preferred treatment tactic at this point in time.

Once a diagnosis has been made and the family has accepted the viability of the diagnosis, the process of functional coping, acceptance, and planning for the future may begin. As discussed earlier in this chapter, coping styles will vary from family member to family member, and may range from active and concerned involvement to emotional detachment and distancing. Acceptance of the situation and the individual with failing memory and cognitive decline will also vary between family members. The role of the therapist at this juncture usually consists of providing support, education, and referral for specific difficulties.

Basic questions concerning financial arrangements, driving ability, or legal issues may arise. Issues around degree of supervision necessary for the individual may occur, and the family may benefit from education concerning the individual's judgment in daily affairs. For example, family members may need guidance concerning medication regimens, inasmuch as the brain-compromised individual may inadvertently fail to take medication as prescribed. Specific family members may react to these needs with a sense of being overwhelmed and demonstrate increased tendencies towards stress-induced irritability and crisis responses to seemingly benign stressors. An empathic, yet empowering consultational stance is ultimately the most beneficial for these family members, as well as for the entire family system. As in the case of traumatic brain injury, the therapist should strive to furnish expert opinion but try to avoid making decisions for the family. The case study below illustrates this approach, as well as several of the other principals involved in dealing with families that face a member with dementia.

Family Study 11.4. The Brookes Family

Joan Brookes was a 76-year-old woman who was widowed for 19 years. A mother of six, Joan had a reputation in the small country community where she lived as being feisty, lovable, and fiercely independent.

Joan had lived alone since her husband died of cancer, eschewing frequent opportunities to move in with any of her willing and highly adoring children. Joan stated her opinion regarding this option matter-of-factly: "Any of my kids that think I'm living with them–again–can forget it."

Fifteen years ago, Joan developed renal failure. She was eventually treated with peritoneal dialysis ("By a very nice doctor") for several years. Later she received a more aggressive "damn hospital dialysis" three times a week when peritoneal dialysis was no longer sufficient. Until the last few months, Joan would drive herself the sixty miles round trip to the dialysis center for the necessary treatments.

Eight months ago, Joan had four instances of becoming extremely disoriented. However, she refused to see a neurologist since "I'm already making one doctor rich enough." Four months ago, she became briefly delusional and finally agreed to a physician's consult. This occurred only after she had twice nearly had an accident on the way to her medical appointments.

Because she remained a diagnostic enigma, Joan was eventually hospitalized "in the nut ward" for further testing. She resisted this strenuously, stating that her Medicare expenses "should be applied to the deficit–not to some old hag like me." Finally, she was successfully pressured by her primary care physician to enter the hospital, much to the complaints of several of Joan's children.

In an inpatient setting it became apparent to the staff and to some of the children that Joan was cognitively impaired and had been covering up her deficits in memory, orientation, and judgment. An eventual diagnosis of "dialysis dementia" was made. A family meeting was called to plan for Joan's discharge.

All six of the children contacted the therapist prior to the meeting. Each expressed their opinions regarding discharge plans for their mother. During the family meeting it became evident that three of the children refused to believe that Joan's problems were severe or permanent. Family tension was extremely high. No viable plans were able to be made. The therapist terminated the meeting and planned for a follow-up session the following week.

Between the two meetings, four of the six children called the therapist to complain about each other or about their mother's quality of care at the hospital.

While talking with the family members, the therapist became convinced that no one in the system wanted to take responsibility for making the decision that Joan could no longer reside alone and should leave her home. Although any of the children would have been more than happy to have Joan live with them, no one wanted the role of deciding this or telling their decision to their mother. Instead, the family seemed to "pull" for having the therapist and Joan's physicians decide her fate for her and for them.

The therapist suspected that Joan was sufficiently strong-willed that she might thwart any decision that did not directly come from her children. Consequently, she refused to let the family credit her or the physicians for any judgment regarding Joan's ability to live independently. She was determined to allow the family to decide this for themselves.

It took four additional meetings with the family for them to make this decision, and two more to decide which family member Joan would live with. During this time, the therapist acted primarily as a consultant, sharing her experiences regarding other elderly patients in similar circumstances, and educating the family on Joan's unique needs. It was very difficult for the therapist to avoid hastening the family's decision making. Although she became frustrated at their sluggishness, she was determined that the family solve their own problems.

With the entire family behind the decision, Joan made a smooth transition to a daughter's residence which was close to the medical center where Joan received dialysis. Joan also agreed to stop driving in exchange for family members transporting her around the neighborhood on weekends.

As with the traumatic brain injury patient, the family must eventually reintegrate the changed individual within the familial unit. Throughout this process, family roles are redefined, as when an adult daughter must supervise an aging parent around use of medication. However, the issue is complicated inasmuch as the dementia is usually progressive and ultimately the individual must be placed in a nursing home or other supervised environment. Hence, the family is confronted with accepting and attempting to reintegrate the individual within the family unit, while simultaneously facing the prospect of placing the individual in an institution.

This chapter has approached families of brain-compromised individuals through use of developmental frameworks that take into account the nature of onset of cerebral dysfunction and other variables. There is much that remains to be explored in this exciting and challenging area of family therapy and crisis intervention, and little is known concerning the positive prognosticators of successful familial and individual adjustment to brain-compromise. However, cognizance of unique difficulties faced by these families yields a promising point of departure in effective implementation of coping, adjustment strategies, and family therapy.

Chapter Twelve

Final Words on Treatment Resistance

This final chapter highlights some rules of thumb regarding treatment of the resistant family. Although these guidelines are not absolute, they are often useful for the clinician. We rank them in no particular order of importance.

1. Do not beg, cajole, or force the resistant family into treatment. Instead, suggest that the crisis at hand will repeat unless the family takes certain positive steps. Then be prepared to understand that the system may not always accept your suggestions. In these situations, put your ego "on the back burner."

2. Do not try to rescue the resistant family from itself. Instead, try to use the system's members to implement proposed interventions. Remember, it's okay to fail, if you choose to do so. That's how we all learn.

3. Do not give the resistant family behavioral tasks to accomplish that it probably cannot complete. This simply undermines the family's sense of confidence and convinces it that it has no control over when it will fail. To fail when you don't choose to do so makes the possibility of family changes seem all the more remote.

4. Do not destablize a family system that is unlikely to return to for treatment. Instead, help point out to the family how their coping styles are dysfunctional. Encourage them to try more helpful coping methods and advocate these changes as part of a Behavioral Contract.

5. Do not allow the resistant family to bargain with you. It's usually never helpful. Stay within a well-determined policy, regardless of the family's "needs." It is rarely therapeutic to "break the frame."

6. Never be disrespectful of the resistant family, even when they are "a royal pain." Given their resources, knowledge, and systemic realities, you might behave in a similar way if you had a similar crisis! Instead, treat *all families* with appropriate warmth but also professionalism even when they choose to disregard your consultation.
7. Access the power of community supports! These include self-help and religious groups. Assess these areas and make ample and appropriate referrals. Remember, community cures more efficiently than therapy.
8. Avoid pessimism, even with the most treatment resistant family. Instead, always emphasize that there is hope, if and when the family takes appropriate actions.
9. Never entertain criticisms of the resistant family's present therapist(s). Instead, encourage the family to discuss these criticisms directly with the appropriate persons involved. (Obviously, an exception is when a therapist is guilty of client abuse.)
10. Be neither overbearing, nor shy in the consultation reiteration. Instead, maintain a stance of appropriate concern, warmth, empathy, but also matter-of-factness. Accept no excuses, but avoid blame and guilt.

Finally, remember that life goes on, largely out of the control of even the most skilled and gifted therapist. The resistant family may return again and again. Each time they may decide to begin the arduous process of family change. Usually, however, they will not. Do not be disheartened. Keep trying gently and do not be discouraged! Even the most dysfunctional systems sometimes see the light.

References

Abraham, F. Abraham R. & Shaw, C. (1991). *A visual introduction to dynamical systems theory for psychologyy*. Santa Cruz, CA: Aerial Press.

Ackerman, N. (1970). *Family therapy in transition*. Boston: Little Brown.

Ackerman, N. (1967). Prejudice and scapegoating in the family. In G. Zuk and I. Boszormenyi-Nagy (Eds.), *Family therapy and disturbed families*. Palo Alto, CA: Science and Behavior Books.

Ackerman, N. (1958). *Psychodynamics of family life: Diagnosis and treatment of family relationships*. New York: Basic Books.

Alexander, J., Waldron, H., Barton, C. & Mas, C. (1989). The minimizing of blaming attributions and behaviors in delinquent families. *Journal of Consulting and Clinical Psychology, 57*, 19-24.

Anderson, C. & Stewart, S. (1983). *Mastering resistance: A practical guide to family therapy*. New York: Guilford.

Angell, R. (1936). *The family encounters the Depression*. New York: Charles Scribner.

Ansbacher, H. & Ansbacher, R. (1956). *The individual psychology of Alfred Adler*. New York: Basic Books.

Asen, K., George, E., Piper, R. & Stevens, A. (1989). A systems approach to child abuse: Management and treatment Issues. *Child Abuse & Neglect, 13*, 45-57.

Atkinson, B. & McKenzie, P. (1987). Family therapy with adolescent offenders: A collaborative treatment strategy. *American Journal of Family Therapy, 15*, 316-325.

Bahr, H. (1988). Family change and the mystique of the traditional family. In L. Bond & B. Wagner (Eds.), *Families in transition: Primary prevention programs that work*. Beverly Hills, CA: Sage.

Barker, G. (1990). Emergency room "repeaters." In J. Hillard (Ed.), *Manual of clinical emergency psychiatry*. Washington, DC: American Psychiatric Association Press.

Barrett, M. , Sykes, C. & Byrnes, W. (1986). A systemic model for the treatment of intrafamily child sexual abuse. *Journal of Psychotherapy and the Family, 2*, 67-82.

Barton, C. et al. (1985). Generalizing treatment effects of functional family therapy: Three replications. *American Journal of Family Therapy, 13*, 16-26.

Bateson, G., Jackson, D., Haley J. & Weakland, J. (1956). Toward a theory of schizophrenia. *Behavioral Science, 1*, 251-261.

Bengelsdorf, H. & Alden, D. (1987). A mobile crisis unit in the psychiatric emergency room. *Hospital and Community Psychiatry, 38*, 662-665.

Bergin, A. (1967). Some implications of psychotherapy research for therapeutic practice. *International Journal of Psychiatry, 3*, 136-150.

Bettmann, O. (1974). *The good old days: They were terrible.* New York: Random House.

Boss, P. (1988). Family stress. In M. Sussman and S. Steinmetz (Eds.), *Handbook of marriage and the family* (2nd ed.) New York: Plenum.

Bloom, B. (1981). Focused single-session therapy: Initial development and evaluation. In S. Budman (Ed.). *Forms of brief therapy.* New York: Guilford Press.

Boszormenyi-Nagy, I. (1985). Commentary, transgenerational solidarity, therapists mandate and ethics. *Family Process, 24,* 454-456.

Boszormenyi-Nagy, I. & Framo, J. (1965). A theory of relationships: Experience and transaction. In I. Boszormenyi-Nagy & J. Framo (Eds.), *Intensive family therapy: Theoretical and practical aspects*; New York: Harper & Row.

Bowen, M. (1978). *Family therapy in clinical practice.* New York: Jason Aronson.

Brendler, J., Silver, M., Haber, M. & Sargent, J. (1989, March). *Explosive families: Breaking the symptomatic cycle.* Paper presented at the annual symposium of the Family Therapy Networker, Washington DC.

Brown, G. (Ed.). (1968). *The multi-problem dilemma: A social research demonstration with multi-problem families.* Metuchen, NJ: The Scarecrow Press.

Brown, J. (1940). *The psychodynamics of abnormal behavior.* New York: McGraw-Hill.

Buchanan, D. & Chasnoff, P. (1986). Family crisis intervention programs: What works and what doesn't. *Journal of Police Science and Administration, 14,* 161-168.

Burford, G. & Casson, S. (1989). Including families in residential work: Educational and agency tasks. *British Journal of Social Work, 19,* 19-37.

Cade, B. (1975). Therapy with low socio-economic families. *Social Work Today, 6,* 142-145.

Cameron, N. & Rychlak, J. (1985). *Personality development and psychopathology: A dynamic approach* (2nd ed.). Boston: Houghton Mifflin Company.

Caplan, G. (1964). *Principles of preventative psychiatry.* New York: Basic Books.

Carr, A. (1989). Countertransference to families where child abuse has occurred. *Journal of Family Therapy, 2,* 87-97.

Carter, B., Papp, P., Silverstein, O. & Walters, M. (1986). The Procrustean bed. *Family Process, 25,* 301-304.

Carter, E. A. & McGoldrick, M. (Eds.). (1980). *The family life cycle: A framework for family therapy.* New York: Gardner Press.

Cavan, R. & Ranck, K. (1938). *The family and the Depression.* Chicago: University of Chicago Press.

Chamberlain, L. (1991). Chaos theory and family functioning. Paper presented at the First Convention of the Society for the Study of Chaos Theory in Psychology, San Francisco, CA, August, 1991.

Clark, T., Zalis, T. & Sacco, F. (1982). *Outreach family therapy.* New York: Aronson.

Coleman, S. (Ed.). (1985) *Failure in family therapy.* New York: Guilford.

Conte, J. (1986). Sexual abuse and the family: A critical analysis. *Journal of Psychotherapy and the Family, 2*, 113-126.

Cornille, T. (1989). Family therapy and social control with incestuous families. *Contemporary Family Therapy*, 11, 101-118.

Dahrendorf, R. (1967). *Essays in the theory of society.* Stanford, California: Stanford University Press.

Dreikurs, R., Corsini, R., Lowe, R. & Sonstegard, M. (1959). *Adlerian family counseling: A manual for counseling centers.* Eugene, OR: University of Oregon Press.

Elkaim, M., Goldber, A. & Goldbeter-Merinfeld, E., (1987). Analysis of the dynamics of a family system in terms of bifurcations. *Journal of Social and Biological Structures, 10*, 21-36.

Ellison, J., Blum, N. & Barsky, A. (1986). Repeat visitors in the psychiatric emergency service: A critical review of the data. *Hospital and Community Psychiatry, 37*, 37-41.

Estrella, J. (1988). Family transitions, cumulative stress and crises. In C. Falicov (Ed.), *Family transitions.* New York: Guilford.

Everstine, D.S. & and Everstine, L. (1983). *People in crisis: Strategic therapeutic interventions.* New York: Brunner/Mazel.

Falicov, C. (1988). Family sociology and family therapy contributions to the family development framework: A comparative analysis and thoughts on future trends. In C. Falicov (Ed.), *Family transitions.* New York: Guilford.

Faller, K. (1988). Decision making in cases of intrafamilial child sexual abuse. *American Journal of Orthopsychiatry, 58*, 121-128.

Fisch, R., Weakland, J. & Segal, L. (1983). *The tactics of change: Doing therapy briefly.* San Francisco; Jossey Bass.

Framo, J. (1982). *Explorations in marital and family therapy: Selected papers of James L. Framo, Ph.D.* New York: Springer.

Framo, J. (1965). Rationale and techniques of intensive family therapy. In I. Boszormenyi-Nagy & J. Framo (Eds.), *Intensive family therapy: Theoretical and practical aspects.* Hagerstown, MD: Harper & Row.

Frank, J. (1961). *Persuasion and healing: A comparative study of psychotherapy.* Baltimore: Johns Hopkins University Press.

Freud, S. (1938). *The basic writings of Sigmund Freud.* New York: Modern Library.

Garbarino, J., Guttman, E., Wilson-Seeley, J. (1986). *The psychologically battered child.* San Francisco: Jossey-Bass.

Geismer, L. & La Sorte, M. (1964). *Understanding the multi-problem family: A conceptual analysis and exploration in early identification.* New York: Association Press.

Giaretto, H. (1989). Community-based treatment of the incest family. *Psychiatric Clinics of North America, 12*, 351-361.

Giaretto, H. (1982). A comprehensive child abuse sexual treatment program. *Child Abuse & Neglect, 6*, 263-278.

Gleick, J. (1987). *Chaos: Making a new science.* New York: Viking.

Goldenberg, I. & Goldenberg, H. (1983). Historical roots of contemporary family therapy. In B. Wolman and G. Stricker (Eds.), *Handbook of family and marital therapy*. New York: Plenum.

Gordon, D., Arbuthnot, J., Gustafson, K. & McGreen, P. (1988). Home-based behavioral-systems family therapy with disadvantaged juvenile delinquents. *American Journal of Family Therapy, 16*, 243-255.

Gray, W. & Rizzo, N. (1969). History and development of general systems theory. In W. Gray, F. Duhl & N. Rizzo (Eds.), *General systems theory and psychiatry*. Boston: Little Brown.

Grunebaum, J. (1987). Multi-directed partiality and the "parental imperative." *Psychotherapy, 24*, 646-656.

Guerin, P. (1976). Family therapy: The first twenty-five years. In P. Guerin (Ed.), *Family therapy: Theory and practice*. New York: Gardner Press.

Gurman, A. & Kniskern, D. (1978). Deterioration in marital and family therapy: Empirical, clinical, and conceptual issues. *Family Process, 17*, 3-20.

Haley, J. (1980). Leaving home: *The therapy of disturbed young people*. New York: McGraw-Hill.

Haley, J. (1976). *Problem-solving therapy*. San Francisco: Jossey-Bass.

Henggeler, S. et al. (1986). Multisystemic treatment of juvenile offenders: Effects on adolescent behavior and family interaction. *Developmental Psychology, 22*, 132-141.

Hill, R. (1949). *Families under stress*. New York: Harper & Row.

Hornblow, A. (1986). The evolution and effectiveness of telephone counseling services. *Hospital and Community Psychiatry, 37*, 731-733.

Jackson, D. (1965). Family rules: Marital quid pro quo. *Archives of General Psychiatry, 12*, 589-594.

Jackson, D. (1957). The question of family homeostasis. *Psychiatric Quarterly Supplement, 31*, 79-90.

Johnson, J. (1989). *The relation of observation of parental violence in family of origin, support network variables, social support, and alcohol abuse in male spouse abusers*. Unpublished doctoral dissertation, Loyola University, Chicago.

Johnson, T. (1978). A contextual approach to treatment of juvenile offenders. *Offender Rehabilitation, 3*, 171-179.

Johnson, T. (1977). The results of family therapy with juvenile offenders. *Juvenile Justice, 28*, 29-34.

Johnson, T. (1974). Hooking the involuntary family into treatment: Family therapy in a juvenile court. *Family Therapy, 1*, 79-82.

Kagan, R., Reid, W., Roberts, S. & Silverman-Pollow, J. (1987). Engaging families of court-mandated youths in an alternative to institutional placement. *Child Welfare, 66*, 365-376.

Kantor, D. & Lehr, W. (1975). *Inside the family: Toward a theory of family process*. San Francisco: Jossey-Bass.

Kaplan, L. (1986). *Working with multiproblem families*. Lexington, MA: Lexington Books.

Kaplan, L. (1984). The "multi-problem" family phenomenon: An interactional perspective. Doctoral dissertation, University of Massachusetts.

Kaslow, F. (1980). History of family therapy in the United States: A kaleidoscopic overview. *Marriage and Family Therapy Review, 3,* 77-111.

Kaufman, E. (1985). Family systems and family therapy of substance abuse: An overview of two decades of research and clinical experience. *The International Journal of the Addictions, 20,* 897-916.

Kaufman, K., Tarnowski, K., Simonian, S. & Graves, K. (1991). Assessing the readability of family assessment self-report measures. *Psychological Assessment, 3,* 697-700.

Keeney, B. (1982). Ecological assessment. In J. Hansen & B. Keeney (Eds.), *Diagnosis and assessment in family therapy.* Rockville, MD: Aspen Systems Corporation.

Kolko, D.J. (1987). Treatment of child sexual abuse: Programs, progress, and prospects. *Journal of Family Violence, 2,* 303-318.

Kottler, J. & Blau, D. (1989). *The imperfect therapist.* San Francisco: Jossey-Bass.

L'Abate, L. (1992). *Programmed writing: A self-administered approach for interventions with individuals, couples and families.* Pacific Grove, CA: Brooks/Cole.

L'Abate, L. (1986). *Systematic family therapy.* New York: Brunner/Mazel.

L'Abate, L., Farrar, J. & Serritella, D. (1992). (Eds.). *Handbook of differential treatments for addictions.* Needham Heights, MA: Allyn and Bacon.

Lambert, M., Bergin, A. & Collins, J. (1977). Therapist-induced deterioration in psychotherapy. In A. Gurman & A. Razin (Eds.), *Effective psychotherapy: A handbook of research.* New York: Pergamon Press.

Landau-Stanton, J. (1990). Issues and methods of treatment for families in cultural transition. In M. Mirkins, (Ed.), *The social and political context of family therapy.* Needham Heights, MA: Allyn and Bacon.

Landau-Stanton, J. & Stanton M.D. (1985). Treating suicidal adolescents and their families. In M. Mirkin & S. Koman (Eds.), *Handbook of adolescence and family therapy.* New York: Gardner Press.

Landau-Stanton, J., Griffiths, J. & Mason, J. (1982). The extended family in transition. Clinical implications. In F. Kaslow (Ed.). *The international book of family therapy.* New York: Brunner/Mazel.

Langsley, D., Pittman, F. & Swank, G. (1969). Family crisis in schizophrenics and other mental patients. *Journal of Nervous and Mental Disease, 149,* 270-276.

Langsley, D. & Kaplan, D. (1968). *The treatment of families in crisis.* New York: Grune & Stratton.

Langsley, D., Pittman, F., Machotka, P. & Flomenhaft, K. (1968). Family crisis therapy: Results and implications. *Family Process, 7,* 145-148.

Larson, N. & Maddock, J. (1986). Structural and functional variables in incest family systems: Implications for assessment and treatment. *Journal of Psychotherapy and the Family, 2,* 27-44.

Lazarus, R. & Folkman, S. (1984). *Stress, appraisal, and coping.* New York: Springer.

Lazarus, R. (1966). *Psychological stress and the coping process.* New York: McGraw Hill.

Lazarus, R. (1984). On the primacy of cognition. *American Psychologist, 39,* 124-129.

Lein, L. (1986). The changing role of the family. In M. Lystrad (Ed.), *Violence in the home: Interdisciplinary perspectives.* New York: Brunner/Mazel.

Lessin, S. & Jacob, T. (1984). Multichannel communication in normal and delinquent families. *Journal of Abnormal Child Psychology, 12,* 369-383.

Levy, J. & McCown, W. (1983, December). *Family therapy as crisis intervention.* Symposium presented at the First Prince William County Family Therapy Conference, Manassas, Virginia.

Lezak, M. (1986). Neuropsychological Assessment (2nd ed.). New York: Oxford University Press.

Lidz, T. (1973). *The origins and treatment of schizophrenic disorders.* New York: Basic Books.

Lidz, T., Cornelison, A., Terry, D. & Fleck, S. (1958). Intra-familial environment of the schizophrenic patient: IV. The transmission of irrationality. *AMA Archives of Neurology and Psychiatry, 79,* 305-316.

Lidz, T., Cornelison, A., Fleck, S. & Terry, D. (1957). The intrafamilial environment of schizophrenic patients. II. Marital schism and marital skew. *American Journal of Psychiatry, 114,* 241-248.

Lipsitt, P. Lelos, D. & Gibbs, M. (1985). A family-oriented alternative to pre-trial detention of juveniles. *American Journal of Family Therapy, 13,* 61-66.

Lombardi, J. (1990). *Failure in family therapy: An investigation of two models.* Unpublished thesis, Hahnemann University.

Maier, S. & Seligman, M. (1976). Learned helplessness: Theory and evidence. *Journal of Experimental Psychology: General, 105,* 3-46.

Marks, T. (1991). The fractal geometry of human nature. Paper presented at the First Convention of the Society for the Study of Chaos Theory in Psychology, San Francisco, CA, August, 1991.

Martin, B. (1977). Brief family intervention: Effectiveness and the importance of including the father. *Journal of Consulting Psychology, 45,* 1002-1010.

Maskin, M. (1976). The differential impact of work-oriented vs. communication-oriented juvenile corrections programs upon recidivism rates in delinquent males. *Journal of Clinical Psychology, 32,* 431-433.

Maynard, P. & Hultquist, A. (1988). The Circumplex Model with adjudicated youths' families. *Journal of Psychotherapy and the Family, 4,* 249-266.

McKown, W. (1990). Impulsivity and twelve-step self-help "success": A prospective study. *British Journal of Addictions, 85,* 635-637.

McCown, W. & Johnson, J. (1992a). *Empirical studies of crisis-prone and treatment resistant families.* Glenside, PA: Psychological Associates, Inc.

McCown, W. & Johnson, J. (1992b). An overview of substance abuse. In P. Sutker and H. Adams (Eds.) *Comprehensive handbook of psychopathology.* New York: Plenum.

McCown, W. & Johnson, J. (1992c). Characteristics of treatment resistant families. Paper presented at the annual meeting of the Eastern Psychological Association, Boston, MA, April, 1992.

McCown, W. & Johnson, J. (1991). *Empirical characteristics of crisis-prone families.* Paper presented at the annual meeting of the American Psychological Association, San Fransisco, California, August, 1991.

McCown, W. & Johnson, J. (1989). *Differential arousal gradients in chronic procrastination.* Paper presented at the annual meeting of the American Psychological Society, Washington, DC.

McCown, W. & Johnson, J. (1985). *Measuring processes involved in decision by probation officers to recommend court ordered psychotherapy.* Paper presented at the meeting for the Society for Criminal Justice Sciences, Las Vegas, Nevada.

McCown, W., Johnson, J. & Austin, S. (1986). Inability of delinquents to decode facial expressions of emotion. *Social Behavior and Personality, 1,* 91-97.

McCubbin, H. & Figley, C. (Eds.), (1983). *Stress and the family. Vol I: Coping with normative transition.* New York: Brunner/Mazel.

Meichenbaum, D. & Turk, D. (1987). *Facilitating treatment adherence: A practitioner's guidebook.* New York: Plenum.

Merton, R. (1968). *Social theory and social structure.* Glencoe, IL: Free Press.

Minuchin, S. (1974). *Families and family therapy.* Cambridge: Harvard University Press.

Minuchin, S. & Montalvo, B. (1967). Techniques for working with disorganized low socioeconomic families. *American Journal of Orthopsychiatry, 37,* 880-887.

Minuchin, S., Rosman, B. & Baker, L. (1978). *Psychosomatic families: Anorexia nervosa in context.* Cambridge, MA: Harvard University Press.

Minuchin, S., Montalvo, B., Guerney, B., Rosman, B. & Schudmer, F. (1967). *Families of slums: An exploration of their structure and treatment.* New York: Basic Books.

Moos, R. & Schaeffer, J. (1986). Life transitions and crises. In R. Moos (Ed.), *Coping with life crisis.* New York and London: Plenum.

Moranze, C. (1957/1966). *The triumph of the middle classes.* New York: Anchor (First published in 1957).

Morganson, P. (1987). *Early renaissance society.* London: Routledge.

Mowrer, E. (1927). *Family disorganization.* Chicago: University of Chicago Press.

Newhill, C. (1989). Psychiatric emergencies: Overview of clinical principles and clinical practice. *Clinical Social Work Journal, 17,* 245-258.

Nezu, A., Nezu, C. & Perri, M. (1989). *Problem-solving therapy for depression: Theory, research and clinical guidelines.* New York: Wiley and Sons.

Nichols, W. (1986). Understanding family violence: An orientation for family therapists. *Contemporary Family Therapy, 8,* 188-207.

Nisbett. R. (1953) *The quest for community*. New York: Oxford University Press.

Nurius, P. (1983-1984). Emergency psychiatric services: A study of changing utilization patterns and issues. *International Journal of Psychiatry in Medicine, 13*, 229-254.

Olson, D. (1970). Marital and family therapy: Integrative review and critique. *Journal of Marriage and the Family, 32*, 501-538.

Olson, D., Portner, J. & Lavee, Y. (1985). *FACES III*. St. Paul: Family Social Science, University of Minnesota.

Olson, D., Russell, C. & Sprenkle, D. (1980). Marital and family therapy. A decade review. *Journal of Marriage and the Family, 42*, 973-993.

O'Shee, M. & Jessee, E. (1982). Ethics, values, and professional conflicts in systems therapy. In J. Hansen & L. L'Abate (Eds.) *Values, ethics and legalities in family therapy*. Rockville, MD. Aspen.

Oster, G. & Caro, J. (1990). *Understanding and treating the depressed adolescents and their families*. New York: Wiley.

Pardeck, J. T. (1989). Family therapy as a treatment approach to child abuse. *Family Therapy, 16*, 113-120.

Parsons, B. & Alexander, J. (1973). Short-term family intervention: A therapy outcome study. *Journal of Consulting and Clinical Psychology, 41*, 196-201.

Parsons, T. (1955). Family structure and the socialization of the child. In T. Parsons & R. Bales (Eds.), *Family, socialization, and interaction process*. New York: The Free Press.

Parsons, T. & Bales, R. (1955). *Family, socialization, and interaction process*. New York: The Free Press.

Paul, G. (1967). Strategy of outcome research in psychotherapy. *Journal of Consulting Psychology, 31*, 109-118.

Perlmutter, R. & Jones, J. (1986). Psychiatric emergency programs. In L. Wynne, S. McDaniel & T Weber (Eds.), *System consultation: A new perspective for family therapy*. New York: Guilford.

Perlmutter, R. & Jones, J. (1985). Assessment of families in psychiatric emergencies. *American Journal of Orthopsychiatry, 55*, 130-139.

Pernett, K. & Urwitz, R. (1990, January). The effects of sexual abuse on its victims: A CYA perspective or reabuse by the system. Presented at the Sexual Abuse Prevention and Education Network–East conference, January 11-12, 1990.

Phares, E. (1992). *Clinical psychology: Concepts, methods, and profession* (2nd ed.). Pacific Grove, CA:Brooks/Cole.

Phillips, E. (1988). *Patient compliance: New light on health delivery systems in medicine and psychotherapy*. Lewiston, NY: Hans Huber.

Pittman, F. (1988). Family crisis: Expectable and unexpectable. In C. Falicov (Ed.), *Family transitions*. New York: Guilford.

Pittman, F. (1987). *Turning points: Treating families in transition and crisis*. New York: Norton.

Pittman, F. (1973). Managing psychiatric emergencies: Defining the family crisis.

In D. Bloch (Ed.), *Techniques of family psychotherapy: A primer*. New York: Grune & Stratton.

Satir, V. (1972). *Peoplemaking*. Palo Alto: Science and Behavior Books.

Satir, V. (1967). *Conjoint family therapy: A guide to theory and technique*. Palo Alto, CA: Science and Behavior Books.

Schlesinger, B. (1963). *The multi-problem family: A review and annotated bibliography*. Toronto: University of Toronto Press.

Seligman, M. & Maier, S. (1967). Failure to escape traumatic shock. *Journal of Experimental Psychology, 74*, 1-9.

Seyle, H. (1956). *The stress of life*. New York: McGraw-Hill.

Sherman, R. & Dinkmeyer, D. (1987). *Systems of family therapy: An Adlerian Integration*. New York: Brunner/Mazel.

Shure, M.B. (1992a). *I Can Problem Solve (ICPS): An Interpersonal Cognitive Problem Solving Program (preschool)*, Champaign, IL: Research Press.

Shure, M.B. (1992b). *I Can Problem Solve (ICPS): An Interpersonal Cognitive Problem Solving program (kindergarten/primary grades)*, Champaign, IL: Research Press.

Shure, M.B. (1992c). *I Can Problem Solve (ICPS): An Interpersonal Cognitive Problem Solving program (intermediate elementary grades)*, Champaign, IL: Research Press.

Singer, M. & Wynne, L. (1965). Thought disorder and family relations of schizophrenics: III. Methodology using projective techniques. *Archives of General Psychiatry, 12*, 187-200.

Solomon, R. (1980). The opponent process theory of acquired motivation: The costs of pleasure and the benefits of pain. *American Psychologist, 35*, 691-712.

Solomon, R. & Corbit, J. (1974). An opponent-process theory of motivation: I. Temporal; dynamics of affect. *Psychological Review, 81*, 119-145.

Stanton, M.D. (1980). Some overlooked aspects of the family and drug abuse. In B.G. Ellis (Ed.), *Drug abuse from the family perspective*. Rockville, MD: NIDA, DHEW.

Stanton, M.D., Todd, T. & Associates (1982). *The family therapy of drug abuse and addiction*. New York: Guilford.

Stanton, M.D. & Todd, T. (1981). Engaging "resistant" families in treatment: II. Principles and techniques in recruitment. *Family Process, 20*, 261-280.

Steinglass, P. (1977). Family therapy in alcoholism. In Kissin, B & Begleiter, H. *The Biology of Alcoholism, vol 5*. New York: Plenum.

Stuart, R. (1980). *Helping couples change: A social learning approach to marital therapy*. New York: Guilford.

Stuart, R., Jayartone, S. & Tripodi, T. (1976). Changing adolescent deviant behavior through reprogramming the behavior of parents and teachers: An experimental evaluation. *Canadian Journal of Behavioral Science, 8*, 132-143.

Sugarman, S. & Masheter, C. (1986). The family crisis intervention literature: What is meant by crisis? *International Journal of Family Psychiatry, 7*, 359-376.

Sutton, L. (1978). *CHIP (Children in Need of Supervision Intervention Project)-A study of juvenile recidivism*. Washington: U.S. Government Printing Office.

Taylor, J. (1986). Social casework and the multimodal treatment of incest. *Social Casework, 67*, 451-459.

Todd, T. (1988). Developmental cycles and substance abuse. In C. Falicov (Ed.), *Family transitions*. New York: Guilford.

Todd, T. & Stanton, M.D. (1983). Research on marital and family therapy: Answers, issues, and recommendations for the future. In B. Wolman and G. Stricker (Eds.), *Handbook of family and marital therapy*. New York: Plenum.

Tolan, P., Cromwell, R. & Brasswell, M. (1986). Family therapy with delinquents: A critical review of the literature. *Family Process, 25*, 619-649.

Tormey, J. (1985). Commentary on Charles Hanly's "Logical and Conceptual Problems of Existential Psychiatry." *Journal of Nervous and Mental Disease, 173*, 276-277.

Trepper, T. (1986). The apology session. *Journal of Psychotherapy and the Family, 2*, 93-101.

Trepper, T. & Sprenkle, D. (1989). The clinical use of the circumplex model in the assessment and treatment of intrafamily child sexual abuse. *Journal of Psychotherapy and the Family, 4*, 93-111.

Trepper, T. & Barrett, M. (1986a). Introduction to the multiple systems perspective for the treatment of intrafamily child sexual abuse. *Journal of Psychotherapy and the Family, 2*, 5-12.

Trepper, T. & Barrett, M. (1986b). Vulnerability to incest: A framework for assessment. *Journal of Psychotherapy and the Family, 2*, 13-26.

Tseng, W. & Hsu, J. (1991). *Culture and family: Problems and therapy*. Binghamton, NY: The Haworth Press.

Ulrici, D. (1983). The effects of behavioral and family interventions on juvenile recidivism. *Family Therapy, 10*, 25-36.

von Bertalanffy, L. (1968). *General systems theory: Foundation, development, applications*. New York: Braziller.

Williams, R. (1976). *Keywords: A vocabulary of culture and society*. New York: Oxford University Press.

Worthington, E. (1987). Treatment of families during life transitions: Matching treatment to family response. *Family-Process, 26*, 295-308.

Zuck, G. (1971). *Family therapy: A triadic-based approach*. New York: Behavioral Publications.

Index

NOTES

NOTES

NOTES

NOTES

NOTES

NOTES

NOTES

NOTES